How to Get into Medical School in Australia

How to Get into Medical School in Australia

The Definitive Guide to Applying to Medical School

Timothy Shiraev

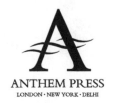

ANTHEM PRESS
LONDON · NEW YORK · DELHI

Anthem Press
An imprint of Wimbledon Publishing Company
www.anthempress.com

This edition first published in UK and USA 2013
by ANTHEM PRESS
75–76 Blackfriars Road, London SE1 8HA, UK
or PO Box 9779, London SW19 7ZG, UK
and
244 Madison Ave. #116, New York, NY 10016, USA

British Library Cataloguing-in-Publication Data
A catalogue record for this book is available from the British Library.

Library of Congress Cataloging-in-Publication Data
How to get into medical school in Australia : the definitive guide
to applying to medical school / Timothy Shiraev.
pages cm
Includes bibliographical references and index.
ISBN-13: 978-0-85728-567-6 (pbk. : alk. paper)
ISBN-10: 0-85728-567-X (pbk. : alk. paper)
1. Medical education–Australia. 2. Medical colleges–Admission–Australia. I. Title.
R831.A6S55 2013
610.71'194–dc23
2013000842

ISBN-13: 978 0 85728 567 6 (Pbk)
ISBN-10: 0 85728 567 X (Pbk)

This title is also available as an eBook.

To my family, for your ongoing optimism, support and belief

To Gabi, for your love and encouragement

This book is dedicated to Joshua Scott-Paul (1983–2011)

Contents

Editors and Contributors

Editors

Gabriella Barclay

Chris Thomas

Contributors

Professor Suzanne Anderson

Professor James Angus

Dr Zorik Avakian

Simon Baume

Elijah Burrows

Dr Catherine Crane

Dr Edward Campion

Associate Professor Andrew Dean

Dr Elspeth Fotheringham

Professor Gordian Fulde

Associate Professor Ray Garrick

Tshinta Hoey

Associate Professor Nigel Hope

Anika Johnston

Michael Shiraev

Emily Sutherland

Most of the contributors listed as medical students in this book are soon to graduate from university, and are likely doctors by the time of publication. Their appropriate qualifications will be updated in the next edition of this book.

Users of this guide are encouraged to check all information with the relevant source. Any suggestions would be very much appreciated, and can be emailed to medicalschoolsaustralia@gmail.com.

1 | Introduction

1) Decide medicine is for you

2) Position yourself:

    a. Optimise marks in high school or university

    b. Obtain extra-curricular experience

3) Study and sit for the entry exams (UMAT or GAMSAT)

4) Prepare and submit your application

5) Prepare for and sit your interview

6) Accept your invitation to medical school

Why You Should Read this Book

The purpose of this book is to provide information on how to successfully apply to medical school at Australian universities, as well as how to excel in medical school. When I first became interested in applying to medical school I found it difficult to get my head around all of the steps associated with gaining entry, such as school marks, GPAs, the UMAT, the GAMSAT, applications, interviews and preferences, not to mention the difference between Bonded, Rural Bonded and Commonwealth Supported Places.

To help you through this process, contained in the following chapters is an explanation of the above topics, and an outline of how and when to navigate this process. There are study tips for optimising your marks at school, university and medical school, as well as several pages of practice questions for the admissions exams (UMAT and GAMSAT) and interview. Also included are quotes from people who have excelled in various parts of the process – people who aced their high school leavers exams, medical students, junior and senior doctors. They describe their experiences, and most importantly provide tips and words of advice.

The last chapter describes each medical school in Australia, the number and type of places available, the location of their rural schools, the focus of the school, the entry requirements, and their contact details. Lastly, the References section includes a list of recommended textbooks and resources for assisting in applying to medical school, as well as textbooks to use whilst in medical school. Those books marked with an asterisk are recommended reading and may give you the edge you need.

What It's Like to Become a Doctor

Becoming a doctor is a long process and takes a lot of hard work and dedication. You will need to work hard throughout high school and/or university, sitting extra exams in your final years. Your medical degree takes between four and six years, and includes a combination of university classes (9am–5pm), hospital rotations (7am till late) as well as study at nights and on weekends. Once you have graduated from medical school, you become an intern. For your internship year, you are assigned to several different medical teams over a number of rotations. Although you are rostered on (usually) between 7am and 4pm, you rarely leave before 6pm. After your internship year you become a resident – which is more of the same, but you are more experienced, may work even longer hours, and have an intern to look after; to mentor, teach and train.

After your first year of residency you can apply for 'training' to allow you to enter a particular specialty, but few are accepted until after their second year. Once you have entered your specialty training program as a registrar, your training will take 4–6 years to complete before you are specialised. During this time, you will work incredibly long hours – there are horror stories of registrars working 120-hour weeks. Upon completing your training, you will become a member of one of the medical colleges (for example, the Royal Australasian College of Surgeons, Royal Australasian College of Physicians, Australian and New Zealand College of Anaesthetists and so on). If you are lucky enough to find a spot in a hospital, you will be called a consultant. So, if you are incredibly hard working, dedicated and lucky, you may be fully trained as a doctor somewhere between the ages of 30 and 35.

At this point, you might be asking 'Why would anyone want to do this?' The answer is, because it's a great life. Spending your life studying something you love, being around colleagues who are equally interested, meeting new people, being in a team environment, and getting to help people day in and day out is incredibly rewarding – some say it is 'a calling'. Although it is hard work, it is such an amazing career that it is all worthwhile; it is physically and mentally demanding, but it will reward you many times over if it is something you are truly interested in. As I will go on to say many times in this book, if medicine interests you, then go for it.

Something to consider is the 'medical student tsunami'. With the recent increase in the number of medical students currently enrolled in Australia, there are not enough internship positions to accommodate these graduates. The intern year is a compulsory year, necessary for official registration in Australia, so it is concerning that around 46 medical school graduates missed out on an internship spot for 2013. Unfortunately, it is international students who are most likely to miss out on an internship position, which may force them to search for internship positions outside of Australia. See AMSA's 'National Internship Crisis Update' at www.amsa.org.au/internship-crisis for more information.

> *'One of our lecturers said it best – medicine is all about people; and if you don't genuinely like talking to people, being with people, dealing with people's problems, then maybe medicine isn't the best choice. But if you do, I can honestly say that there's nothing I'd rather be doing, so go for it and don't be disheartened if it doesn't work out first go – there are plenty of pathways into the degree and the more conviction you have that this is what you want to do the better!'*
>
> Anika Johnston, High Distinction Student, Sixth Year Medicine, University of New South Wales

> *'Be very sure of your motivation for doing medicine. If you really love humanity, medicine will never cease to reward you. It is not about achieving status or wealth for yourself. It is a career of service to others, in which paradoxically you will be putting yourself in a humble position as you assist patients, while in the eyes of the community and your patients you will be highly esteemed. Walk humbly, and the career of medicine will be a precious jewel in your life.'*
>
> Associate Professor Andrew Dean, Consultant Emergency Physician, St John of God Hospital, Ballarat

There are many areas into which you can specialise once you graduate from medical school (see Chapter 11: 'You've Made It into Medical School' for more). These include but are not limited to:

- Anaesthesia
- Dermatology
- Emergency medicine
- General practice
- Internal medicine – subspecialties include:
  - Cardiology
  - Clinical pharmacology
  - Dermatology
  - Endocrinology
  - Gastroenterology
  - Geriatric medicine
  - Haematology
  - Immunology
  - Infectious disease
  - Oncology
  - Nephrology (Renal)
  - Neurology
  - Paediatrics
  - Palliative medicine
  - Rheumatology
- Medical administration
- Obstetrics and gynaecology
- Occupational medicine
- Ophthalmology
- Pathology
- Psychiatry
- Public health
- Radiology
- Rehabilitation medicine
- Surgery – the surgical sub-specialties include:
  - Cardiothoracic
  - Neurosurgery
  - Orthopaedics
  - Head and neck
  - Paediatric
  - Plastic and reconstructive
  - Urology
  - Vascular

An additional career path is academia. This can include medical research or teaching, or both. Researchers and clinical teachers are essential to the progress of medicine, and as said by Professor James Angus, dean of Melbourne Medical School, 'Without them there is no future for medical schools or clinical research in Australia'. As you can see from the list above, there are many choices, and there is something for everyone!

Summary of the Application Process

This summary gives you a run-down of the whole process – your pre-medical study (high school or university), the application, medical school and all that happens afterwards. Below are two flow charts to assist you in understanding this process.

First, your marks must be great. This is for many the hardest part, but don't be deterred if they're not, as anything is possible if you're willing to work for it.

In your last year of high school you can sit the medical entrance test called the UMAT (Undergraduate Medicine and Health Sciences Admission Test), or if you are at university you can sit the medical entrance test called the GAMSAT (Graduate Medical School Admissions Test). These take quite a bit of study and preparation. If you are smart enough and lucky enough to score well, you can apply to the universities of your choice. This involves sending an application form, proof of your good marks and often a résumé, an essay on why you want to study medicine and other bits and pieces. If you are lucky enough to receive an invitation to an interview, you will need to prepare for it and afterwards you will need to patiently wait to find out if:

1) Your school or university marks will be good enough to allow you in; and

2) You have passed the interview and have been offered a place in the medicine course at your chosen university.

Although it sounds daunting, remember this process occurs over a year (or more), so don't be disheartened! If medicine is something you really want to do, then go for it and don't give up until you get in. A must-read is the Australian Medical Students' Association (AMSA) website on entry to medical schools (at www.amsa.org.au/content/premed-amsa).

Undergraduate Entry

This process begins in your last year of high school. However, remember that performing extra-curricular activities before your final year gives you more time to achieve them, as well as taking pressure off in your final year.

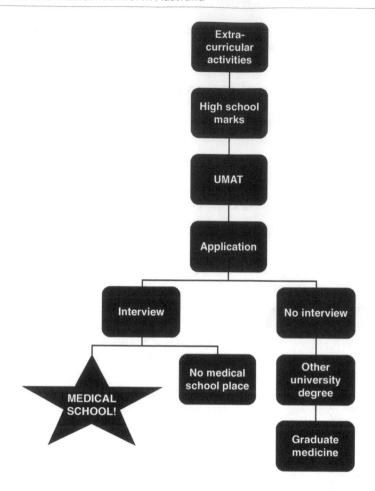

During your last year of high school, you must perform well in your high school marks (see Chapter 3: 'Study Techniques'), sit the UMAT exam (see Chapter 5: 'Undergraduate Entry into Medical School and the UMAT'), and perform extra-curricular activities which look good on your application and in your interview (see Chapter 8: 'The Application'). You must then apply to the universities of your choice. If your high school and UMAT marks are adequate, you will be offered an interview (see Chapter 9: 'The Interview'), after which, if you succeed you will be offered a place in medical school. If you are not successful at any of these points you will not get an offer – in this case, enrol in another university degree and apply for graduate medicine (see the diagram below).

Graduate Entry

During your final 3 years at university, you must perform well in your studies (see Chapter 3: 'Study Techniques'), and if possible complete some extra-curricular activities (see Chapter 8: 'The Application'). In your last or second last year, you must sit the GAMSAT (see Chapter 6: 'Graduate Entry into Medical School and the GAMSAT'), and once your GAMSAT marks have been released, submit an application to your preferred medical school (see Chapter 8: 'The Application'). If your university and GAMSAT marks are adequate, you will be offered an interview (see Chapter 9: 'The Interview') at which if you succeed you will be offered a place in medical school.

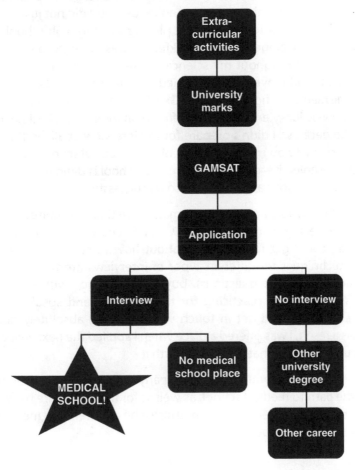

If you are not successful at any of these points, you will not get an offer – in this case, you have several options:

1) Apply again the next year (possibly re-sitting the GAMSAT to improve your mark and gaining more extra-curricular experience)

2) Commence another university degree (either for a different career or in order to improve your university marks so you may reapply for medicine)

3) Try again later – as a mature-aged student

4) Commence a different career

My Experience

My name is Tim Shiraev, and I am an intern at St George Hospital in Sydney. Although I loved every minute of my medical degree, I did not just breeze into medical school. I spent too much time playing sport in high school and as a result got a very average mark – thankfully it was enough to get me into a science degree. Throughout my science degree (and initially without much dedication) I found I loved all of my medical science subjects, so in my final year I sat the medical school entry test (GAMSAT), applied to one of the medical schools and was lucky enough to be offered an interview. I had heard that it was easy to get in so I didn't prepare for my interview at all, and no surprise (looking back on it now), I didn't get an offer to medical school. I was crushed, but knew I deserved it – getting into medical school is definitely not easy and you have to give it your all if you want to be successful.

I re-thought my whole approach and made sure that I optimised each of my steps (my university marks, my GAMSAT mark, and my interview) – reading everything I could get my hands on about how to study at university and interview techniques for different types of interviews (from how to dress to how to answer difficult questions), buying every book with GAMSAT-style questions I could find, practicing for the interview and speaking to every medical student I could get in touch with – leaving absolutely nothing to chance. As a result, I was offered a place when I applied the next year and have never doubted that all that work was worth it.

As a result I decided to write this book for anyone who does not know how to start on the path to medical school, as well as for those who are halfway there but want to optimise their chances, or those who are already in medical school but want to know how best to study.

2 | Characteristics of a Doctor

Q: How do they choose medical students out of the thousands of applicants?

A: *They select students that would make good doctors.*

Q: Then what characteristics make a good doctor?

A: *The answer to this question is easy. Just ask yourself, what is it that doctors do everyday? They interact with patients, patients' families, hospital staff, and take a lead role in solving problems. From this basic (and limited) description alone, we can see that a good doctor would need to be very skilled at communication, teamwork, leadership, and problem solving. This is a good start, but there are other equally important characteristics possessed by good doctors, and therefore, characteristics that the universities seek in medical school applicants. This chapter will discuss the qualities sought in aspiring medical students, why these attributes are important and how to best demonstrate them to your future medical school during the application process and interview.*

Academic Qualities

First of all, doctors need to be intelligent – the academic requirements for medicine are the most stringent of all courses and careers. The hurdles thrown at you to assess your academic ability are high cut-offs for school or university marks and the medical entry tests. Neither of these are perfect indicators of medical school performance or medical competence (Wilkinson 2008), but they are part of the criteria nevertheless. The Undergraduate Medicine and Health Sciences Admissions Test (UMAT) is the entry test for students who have not yet completed a degree, generally sat by high school students. The Graduate Australian Medical School Admissions Test (GAMSAT) is for those who have already been to university, and have a bachelor's degree. They are both held once a year. Further details on the UMAT and the GAMSAT are found in Chapters 4 to 6.

'Spending time in the hospital is my favourite part of medical school, especially at the children's hospital, as it is always changing and there are endless possibilities to learn more about medicine.'

Emily Sutherland, High Distinction Student, Sixth Year Medicine, University of New South Wales

Empathy

For a long time, academic prowess was the only selection criteria considered when choosing prospective medical students. For an equally long time, doctors have been criticised for lacking good 'bedside manner', that is, lacking emotional interest in their patients. As such, it was suggested that doctors be more caring about their patients – not only because this is what we expect of our health professionals, but also because good doctor–patient communication is associated with improvements in patient health (Stewart 1995). The solution was thought to be to select medical students that are more sympathetic towards other people. However, it was soon discovered that sympathy is easy to fake (for example, just saying 'Oh, the poor patient with their sore throat/ weak heart/arthritic joint' rather than actually believing it), as well as the problem that 'sympathy can be burdensome and emotionally exhausting and can lead to burnout' (Hardee 2003).

'I really enjoy my patients. Every encounter is different and seeing patients getting better gives one such a sense of achievement and is very rewarding.'

Dr Elspeth Fotheringham, General Practitioner, Tuggerah

What we actually want from our doctors is not just one who is compassionate, but who can put themselves in the patient's shoes, and care about the patient because they are engaged with them emotionally. As such, empathy is one of the main attributes sought after in prospective medical students (the distinction between sympathy and empathy is discussed by James Hardee in his 2003 article). Some people are naturally more empathic than others – sorry guys, females have been shown to be more empathic (Hojat 2002) – but empathy is widely considered to be a 'learnable' trait. That is, if you don't find yourself to be particularly empathic, this is something you can improve on:

1. Ask yourself 'How would I feel if that happened to me?' If you're still not sure how the other person is feeling, ask them with an open-ended question (a question that requires more than a yes/no answer), such as 'Tell me more about how you are feeling?' or 'How do you feel about your current situation?'

2. Once you've imagined how the patient might be feeling, let them know. For example, 'You must be feeling upset', or 'I can see how that would make you feel frightened'. This lets the patient know you understand how they feel. Or, if you've misinterpreted how the patient is feeling, they will correct you but they will also be thankful that you're trying to understand their situation

3. Lastly, see what you can do to help. It isn't enough just to understand how they feel, you should also do something about it. Importantly, you should let the patient know that you will work with them to solve the problem.

This is a lifetime skill that is worth practicing at home (with friends and family), and trying to integrate into your everyday life. Whether you have a family member upset about something, or a restaurant customer annoyed that their food is late, letting them know that you understand how they feel and that you empathise with them is a great comfort, as well as more likely to reach a good outcome.

> 'The thing I like most about medicine is how it intertwines science (which has always fascinated me) with people (who are also endlessly interesting). As much as I enjoy learning about science, I could never be a scientist working in a lab because my favourite part of medicine is really hearing people's stories and having the privilege of being given a window into their world. The capacity to make a difference to people's lives is another enticing thing about the profession.'
>
> Anika Johnston, High Distinction Student, Sixth Year Medicine, University of New South Wales

The ability to be empathic is incredibly important for admission to medical school – and for being a successful doctor. The empathy of potential medical students is examined during the UMAT and the interview for undergraduates, and at the interview only for graduates.

Communication

Effective communication involves talking openly and honestly, ensuring both parties have complete understanding. In a profession like medicine, not following instructions exactly can have severe repercussions. Flawless communication not only ensures doctors and patients interact effectively, but also that healthcare professionals interact well together, ensuring instructions on patient care are carried out properly. Good communication skills are essential, as whether you are a first year medical student or experienced consultant, you will be communicating with patients, their families, other doctors and other health professionals. As such, communication is one of the most important characteristics possessed by a doctor, and so one of the most heavily examined. In fact, along with assessing empathy, assessing a student's communication skills is one of the reasons interviews were introduced into the selection process. In addition, good communication requires empathy, as it is only by being able to understand how the other person is feeling that you can respond appropriately. See Chapter 8: 'The Application' for activities that both look good on your application and help you learn communication skills.

Teamwork

Teamwork gives the chance for people from different backgrounds and experiences to come together as a group and work towards a common goal. It is crucial for doctors to work effectively in a group situation, whether this be with patients, other doctors, nurses, physiotherapists, social workers, dieticians, dentists, orderlies, psychologists, and the list goes on. For optimal patient care, doctors need input from other health professionals, since no one holds all the answers. As such you need to combine the wisdom and experience of many different professionals, and so be able to work with others efficiently and effectively.

This is especially true for complex cases. For example, if a teenager presents with a drug overdose you need to immediately treat the medical problems (which will most likely involve other doctors) while working alongside the nurses, possibly involving drug and alcohol specialists (who may or may not be medically qualified), and possibly contact a social worker or psychologist to deal with the social and psychological aspects of the patient's illness. Good teamwork relies heavily on good communication, as it is impossible to coordinate and work as a group if you do not have effective communication skills.

Being good at teamwork, being a team player and enjoying being part of a team are a main focus in the medical school selection process (both in the application and at the interview). It is important for you to identify team or group situations that you have been a part of and to identify what role you played in this team or group.

A list of possible team situations that are helpful not just to look good on your application or in the interview, but also to help you learn effective team skills are listed in Chapter 8: 'The Application'.

Leadership

Along with empathy, communication and teamwork, leadership completes the four most important characteristics of a doctor and are the characteristics sought out by interviewers. All members of a healthcare team are essential to optimal healthcare, and the doctor takes the lead. The doctor's role is to provide the focal point for care, overseeing and ensuring there is continuity of care, and coordinating the other health professionals. A good leader in any situation is responsible, leads by example and treats all team members equally.

Leaders need to be good communicators, both with other individuals, and in helping the group communicate as a whole. They must be able to motivate and coordinate the group, and remain calm and level headed in stressful situations. The leader also ensures there is an agreed plan, which has assigned tasks and deadlines, and agreed roles. Good leadership in a doctor is especially important in emergencies as someone has to be in charge – processing all available information, getting input from other professionals and ultimately acting decisively in the best interest of the patient. Medical emergencies require a doctor to respond quickly, confidently and correctly in the given circumstances as there is rarely time for debate about the correct approach. Good leadership also gives confidence to the patient, their family and the other professionals involved in the patient's care.

Leadership qualities of an aspiring medical student are assessed both during the application process and at the interview. As such, it is important you have examples of not only leadership positions you have held, but also how and why you were successful in this role. A list of leadership positions you can put yourself in are listed in Chapter 8: 'The Application'. However, if you have not held any leadership positions, explore the characteristics about yourself that would make you a good leader if given the opportunity.

'I enjoy medicine for a few reasons:

I have always enjoyed helping people in any way that I can, and I chose medicine because I felt that there was no greater way of helping my fellow countrymen than by positively impacting on their health. Nothing can give me greater satisfaction than this. I have always appreciated the care and help I received the many times I have been in hospital. Medicine is a way I can give something back to the community.

Orthopaedics, the career path I have chosen, allows me to help patients return back to near normal function and relieve them of the symptoms of numerous orthopaedic conditions. Helping patients return to a pre-morbid level of function produces a great sense of accomplishment and satisfaction that is addictive in every sense.

Medicine also allows you to interact with a wide variety of cultures and personalities which enriches one's own culture and experiences in life. Medicine is what makes my life complete and without it, I don't feel I would be who I am today.'

Dr Zorik Avakian, Orthopaedic Registrar

Conflict Resolution

A very important characteristic of a good leader which is heavily examined in medical school applicants is the skill of conflict resolution. Interacting in stressful situations with patients, their families, and medical staff on a daily basis means conflict often arises, and often it is up to the leader of the healthcare team to resolve it. Even if you are not in a leadership position you will encounter conflicts and will need to be familiar with the process of conflict resolution. Whether this is conflict within the healthcare team or your personal conflict with another individual, it is important you are comfortable in dealing with issues as they arise.

Questions on conflict resolution are common in most interviews, and are almost certain to be in your medical school interview. A good leader will address any conflict immediately and directly by identifying the source of conflict and then facilitating or mediating a discussion between the conflicting parties. They would then try to reach some kind of agreement, ideally a compromise (see the paper on conflict resolution written for junior doctors: Saltman 2006).

It is important to note that good communication skills and empathy are also important in facilitating conflict resolution.

Self-Reflection

It is important to be introspective prior to your medical school interview and attempt to address any characteristics that may impede your chances of not only gaining entry into medical school but to becoming a successful doctor.

As I was unprepared for my first medical school interview, I did not consider that the interviewer would be assessing whether I possessed the necessary characteristics of a doctor. Although it is in my nature to be shy, I also assumed that I knew how to fake confidence. Upon being rejected that year, I sought out friends and family to give me feedback on areas that may have held me back. The resounding answer was to address my shyness. I started making a conscious effort to be more outgoing at parties and when meeting new people, situations that I normally would have been a bit awkward in. Additionally, I got a job as an orderly (assisting in patient care at a hospital) at a hospital the following year. In this role I met hundreds of staff that I would be interacting with daily, and met new patients day in and day out. Initially this was daunting, however after a month of initial shyness, I started to gain confidence and became more outgoing. Years on, my friends and family are still impressed by the change in me.

No matter how severe your fear of meeting or interacting with new people, your trouble communicating or leading or your lack of empathy, you must realise that as a doctor you will be meeting, communicating, leading and interacting with new people all the time and must feel comfortable and confident while doing so. Not only will this come across to the interview panel, it will make you a better and more competent doctor.

3 | Study Techniques

1) *Decide medicine is for you*

2) **Position yourself:**

   a. ***Optimise marks in high school or university***

   b. *Obtain extra-curricular experience*

3) *Study and sit for the entry exams (UMAT or GAMSAT)*

4) *Prepare and submit your application*

5) *Prepare for and sit your interview*

6) *Accept your invitation to medical school*

Having effective study techniques is essential to getting good marks, getting into medical school and succeeding in medical school. No matter how naturally intelligent you are, there are others that are just as smart as you, but who may be working harder than you. Also, there are people who aren't as smart as you, are working harder – and with hard work will be able to do just as well, if not better than you. So, it's good to get into productive and efficient study habits early on.

Below are study tips for high school and university. Different study techniques may work better for you than others, but it is worthwhile trying anything to improve your study. In medicine, the more you know the better doctor you will be, and it is the same with study techniques – the more tricks and tactics you have up your sleeve, the better studier you will be.

It is essential that while you are optimising your high school or university marks you are also performing extra-curricular activities which will demonstrate that you are a well-rounded high achiever, and therefore demonstrate the characteristics sought in doctors mentioned earlier in the book. These include leadership, teamwork and communication skills, academic ability, and the willingness to give to the community. Some examples include learning a language, playing a team sport, volunteering with children, or joining a debating team. More examples and suggestions on how best to do this are found in Chapter 8: 'The Application'.

How to Study at High School

To achieve good marks, you must stick to a good study plan, as well as having plenty of sleep. A study plan or schedule outlines when and what you will be studying. For example:

0900 – 1500	School
1500 – 1530	Travel home and afternoon tea
1530 – 1620	English study
1620 – 1630	*Break*
1630 – 1720	Physics study
1720 – 1730	*Break*
1730 – 1820	Maths study
1820 – 1900	Dinner
1900 – 1950	Drama study
1950 onwards	Relax and bed

If you have a schedule, you can organise how much time you will be spending on each subject, and ensure you don't study some subjects and neglect others. Also, a schedule including a 'time line' will motivate you to stick to the plan, and you will be less likely to procrastinate. However it is important to remember that a plan is only a guideline and will continually change from day to day and week to week as you will naturally take longer studying some subjects. Keep in mind, you cannot study for hours at a time and continue to learn effectively. You should take 5 to 10 minute breaks every hour or so to keep your brain fresh. Putting this time aside will also ensure that you reduce the amount of time you procrastinate during study times.

'The main thing I found hard about studying in high school was maintaining constant discipline in keeping on top of my workload. It's hard to be disciplined about study because only you can make yourself sit down, read and make notes day after day…without losing your mind. At the end of the day, most people are not very disciplined. So if you can stay disciplined about reaching your goals you are already miles ahead of the pack.

I found the trick to staying disciplined was to 1) Set realistic but challenging goals and 2) Take regular, relaxing breaks.

It was lame, I admit, but I wrote down the UAI (ATAR) and uni course I was aiming for on a piece of paper and hung that piece of paper above where I studied – it made it hard to forget what all my hard work was for!

After studying for an intense period, it didn't matter what I did to relax, as long as it was something completely different to studying. This is how I stayed disciplined (and sane).'

Michael Shiraev, 99.75 UAI (now ATAR) in 2006, Law Student, University of Sydney

There is no one way of studying that works for everyone, but the general rule is: the longer you're sitting in your study chair, the better you will do. Admittedly, it is possible to sit in your chair and procrastinate, play on the internet, Facebook, play games and do anything except study. However, as long as you're sitting at your desk studying effectively, you are increasing your chances of getting good marks.

It has long been known that the more involved with your learning you are, the more you remember. For example, you will remember 10 percent of the text you read, 20 percent of information you hear, 70 percent if you participate in a discussion or give a talk, and 90 percent if you give a presentation, or simulate the actual experience (Mariotti 2009).

'The best way to study in high school is short periods (1 hour) of intense, no-BS study, changing subject each period (hour), with enjoyable, meaningful leisure activities after each period. This allows you to accurately gauge your efforts, reward them, and keep things as interesting as possible.'

Simon Baume, 100 UAI (now ATAR) in 2006, Law Student, University of Sydney

Suggested study techniques include:

* <u>Make summaries of your school work as you go</u>. Highlight the important parts of your notes taken in class, and then make a summary of this. You can then use these summaries as a resource for exam study.
* <u>Use diagrams, pictures and different colours</u> (pens, highlighters, paper, etc.) if you are a visual learner.

- <u>Read textbooks on the subject before it is covered in class</u> and make notes on this so you already have an idea about it before it is discussed (see 'University Study' below for more on this).

- <u>Use flashcards</u>. These are great for remembering formulas, or simple lists. Write the question on one side of a card (the card about the size of your palm), and then write the answer on the reverse side and test yourself. For example:

<u>FRONT</u>	<u>BACK</u>
Formula for **Compound Interest**	$A = P(1+r)^n$ A = final balance P = initial quantity r = percentage rate compounding (decimal) n = number of periods

- <u>Record yourself reading the material and listen to the recording</u>. For example, record it straight onto your iPod.

- <u>Repeat or explain topics out loud</u>. Whether explaining to others (for example friends or family) or just talking out loud to yourself, this can reinforce a subject in your mind.

- <u>Study in a group</u>. Teaching other people helps to consolidate your knowledge and points out your weaker areas. Just make sure you don't distract each other!

- <u>Focus on weak areas</u>. You may enjoy studying areas you are confident in, but your weaker areas will benefit more from time spent studying.

> 'In high school, it is important to get a mix of quiet study on your own – reading your texts, making notes and mind maps and doing practice papers – as well as group study with other smart and hard working students. You need to put in the hours by yourself to understand the basics, but difficult concepts will sometimes only make sense after some lively group discussion. Look out for the disciplined students around you and try to learn from them and with them.'
>
> Michael Shiraev, 99.75 UAI (now ATAR) in 2006, Law Student, University of Sydney

'*I would advise students to select a broad range of subjects, as it will prepare them well for university and the outside world. It also helps students better identify what they are interested in and what may be a likely career path for them.*

Tips would be:

– *Always do more than what is recommended in terms of exercises and reading*

– *Work hard consistently throughout the HSC years*

– *Do lots of practice and past paper questions.*'

Dr Zorik Avakian, Orthopaedic Registrar

• <u>Be up to date with each topic</u>. Do not move on until you have complete understanding of each topic. Learning is cumulative – everything is built upon something else you have already learnt. For example, you learn anatomy and physiology (how the body works when it is healthy) before learning pathology (how the body works when it is sick). If you don't understand something, or are having trouble with a particular concept, ask someone, or do some more research on it yourself. Keep a list of the things you do not understand and make sure you address these areas.

• <u>Use mnemonics</u>. Medical students have been using mnemonics for years to help them remember things. A mnemonic is a group of letters or ideas that helps your memory. For example, a well-known way to remember the symptoms of depression is SAD-A-FACES (Ellen 1997), which stands for <u>S</u>leep change, <u>A</u>ppetite change, <u>D</u>ysphoria (bad mood), <u>A</u>nhedonia (loss of interest in fun things), <u>F</u>atigue, <u>A</u>gitation, <u>C</u>oncentration problems, <u>E</u>steem problems, and <u>S</u>uicidal thoughts – see how it would be impossible to remember these things in a random order, but remembering SAD-A-FACES lets you remember them all easily? You will hear many mnemonics during your degree, but feel free to make them up yourself. If you find you can't remember a list of things, try taking the first letter of each thing and make a word with them all – you'll never forget the list then!

'Study with friends and quiz each other – this will be the stuff you really remember! Also, utilise school resources such as the library or study sessions with teachers, and don't be afraid to ask questions if you don't understand anything. Often teachers will also be willing to stay back after school or help you during lunch if you're really struggling with something.'

Emily Sutherland, High Distinction Student, Sixth Year Medicine, University of New South Wales

Many high schools organise study skills workshops run by outside companies, which are extremely helpful for all students. Enquire at your school if one is planned for your year group, or request for one to be organised. A well-known company is Elevate Education (see the References section for details).

Exam Study

I recommend starting to revise long before your exams. This will help to point out your weaker areas and will give you time to do the necessary research required (including self study, meeting with your teacher or friend) to understand those areas. It will also give you time to consolidate and build upon what you know with time free for practice papers and questions. The last minute, frantic scramble to cram doesn't work. Some people manage to get good marks doing this, but they could do even better if they studied for exams thoroughly, over a longer time frame, and then would be more likely to retain that knowledge.

'There is no way that you can cram everything for exams. It makes life a lot easier if you consistently work away at it (easy for me to say, having been forced to study at boarding school).

Also, engage in class and make the most out of the structured teaching. This is a big one. Why bother spending hours trying to understand some concept in a textbook if there is someone being paid to explain it to you in person? Instead of sitting in class and waiting for the period to end, listen to the teacher, engage and ask questions. It will save you so much time and make everything easier to learn.

Choose subjects you enjoy, it will make listening and studying so much easier. Who cares if 4 unit maths scales better than visual arts or PE, if you *find math boring and would enjoy the other subjects? If you blitz one of the lower scaling subjects then you will end up with a great mark. If you struggle in a high scaling subject then you will do poorly.'*

Dr Ed Campion, Intern, St Vincent's Hospital, Sydney

Studying for exams is slightly different from studying during the year. If you haven't done any work during the year, then pre-exam study involves you trying to learn a whole year's worth of content. If you have studied during the year, then the information is already in your brain, and you just need to revise to make sure that you remember everything correctly. Just like studying during the year (see above), it is helpful to construct an exam study timetable.

Exam study differs for everyone, but here are a few general tips:

- Read the notes you made from the textbook. These will re-introduce you to the topic.

- Read the summaries you made from your class notes. These will remind you of important concepts and help cement things in your mind.

- Make a shorter summary of your summaries. Think of it as distilling your notes until you have a great new set of very concentrated notes.

- Study in groups. Each person will have strengths and weaknesses in different areas, and this is a great way to learn – since the best way to learn is to teach! Others might have a good way of explaining a concept, or have a good mnemonic (see above for more on mnemonics) to help you remember a concept.

- Complete practice questions. Practice questions are invaluable, whether past papers or just questions similar to those you think they will be asking. Use them before you begin studying to ensure you are on the right track and/or just prior to the exam, once you have acquired as much knowledge as you can, and see if you can apply it.

- Keep using the notes and aids you made earlier in the year (see above), like your flash cards, and recordings of your voice.

- Ask someone to test you out aloud. This will give you a good indication of what you do and do not know.

- Ask for help from a teacher or friend if you are having trouble with learning or studying effectively. There are also many books and websites on studying in high school (see http://hsc.csu.edu.au/study/ for more information), and on how to study for individual subjects.

> **Q:** What are your tips for optimising high school marks?
>
> **A:** *'Practice papers. Do every one – trial and final – that you find. Do them twice, under exam conditions. And check your answers!*
>
> *Make a list of things you learn from each paper.'*
>
> Simon Baume, 100 UAI (now ATAR) in 2006, Law Student, University of Sydney

> *'Summarise then memorise.'*
>
> Associate Professor Nigel Hope, Consultant Orthopaedic Surgeon, Sydney Adventist Hospital

> *'To maximise high school marks, do more papers and go through the answers with your teachers. When your teachers offer to mark your practice papers, actually take them up on their offer.'*
>
> Michael Shiraev, 99.75 UAI (now ATAR) in 2006, Law Student, University of Sydney

How to Study at University

Studying effectively at university is different to learning in high school because you are given less guidance and direction. At university the number of lectures you go to and the number of tutorials you participate in is up to you and the only consequence of not attending is your own disadvantage. Therefore at university you need to be more dedicated and motivated to stay on top of your work to achieve your goals.

In addition you will have an increased workload and a greater number of assignments, reports and presentations. It is important to be organised with a diary or calendar so that you are prepared prior to due dates. This way, you give yourself plenty of warning when things are due, will have plenty of time to get assignments prepared and plenty of time to study for exams. A semester plan may include your assessments, when they are due, how much they are worth, as well as when you plan to start studying for or preparing them.

'Be organised. Plot your assessments on a calendar and start them early. Attend everything. Many students become lazy throughout the semester and skip classes. Don't fall into this trap.'

Dr Ed Campion, Intern, St Vincent's Hospital, Sydney

The recommendations for studying at university are as per those recommendations for studying at school (see above). The main focus is to be prepared before you attend your lectures by:

- Making notes on that topic from textbooks before attending your lecture. Many lecturers assume you have done this prior to each class although very few people (if any) do. Textbooks have multiple authors and editors so are generally well written, plus have great pictures and diagrams that help illustrate their point – in a way that the lecturer or tutor might not be able to.

- Making summaries of your lectures immediately after you have had them. Retention of knowledge decreases exponentially, from close to 90 percent retention in the hour following the lecture, to 30 percent in 24 hours, to 10 percent within three to six days (Fritz 2011). Also add any additional information from the lecture into these notes.

These notes, written in your own words, can then be used as your study notes for exams. This process will concrete the information in your mind, increasing your retention of the information and ensuring that by the time exams are close you will be prepared with well written and comprehensive study notes.

Often university subjects have a set of criteria that they use as a teaching guide. Use these criteria as subheadings for your notes/summaries. This way, you know exactly what they expect from you and are able to apply your knowledge exactly as they want you to be able to.

'Medicine is first and foremost about people – don't forget how to communicate by burying yourself under a mountain of books for 6 months!'

Anika Johnston, High Distinction Student, Sixth Year Medicine, University of New South Wales

Other study techniques include those mentioned in 'High School Study', such as palm cards, recording information onto your iPod and group study sessions.

Exam Study

At university the last minute, frantic scramble to cram does not work. Although you may manage to get good marks by doing this, your retention of the information is reduced. In addition, university subjects are cumulative and if you do not have a firm and concrete understanding of the basics this will set you back in years to come.

Refer to 'Exam Study' in High School Study Techniques above for tips on how to prepare for exams.

4 | Overview on Applying to Medical School

1) *Decide medicine is for you*

2) **Position yourself:**

   a. **Optimise marks in high school or university**

   b. **Obtain extra-curricular experience**

3) **Study and sit for the entry exams (UMAT or GAMSAT)**

4) **Prepare and submit your application**

5) *Prepare for and sit your interview*

6) *Accept your invitation to medical school*

The challenge in applying to medical school is to ensure you balance this (studying, sitting medical entry tests, writing applications and preparing for interviews) with your current schedule. Often interviewees misrepresent themselves by being unprepared, so it is important to balance your current study with the much needed preparation and study for applying to medical school. It is important to remember that application forms are due at various times throughout the year (generally anywhere from May to September), so check your preferred medical school's website for specific dates.

This chapter contains a guide to when to start studying for your entry tests, when to start preparing for interviews and what to expect along the way.

> *'Making life-long friends has been a major bonus during uni. It is great to have close uni friends to lean on when experiencing the hardships of medical school, such as witnessing a death, or hearing a patient has a terminal illness.'*
>
> Emily Sutherland, High Distinction Student, Sixth Year Medicine, University of New South Wales

It is important to keep in mind that there are many ways to enter medical school, and if you are rejected once, your chances of succeeding the next time are improved as you are already familiar with the process. Undergraduate and graduate medical schools both have their benefits and drawbacks (see below). In addition, the number of places in medical schools has increased markedly over the past few years and will continue to increase (Joyce 2007) – improving your chances of getting a spot in medical school.

If you are not successful at achieving the result required to get into medicine, do not be disheartened as there are other methods for gaining entry into a medical degree. What is important is that you enrol in another degree which gives you a 'foot in the door' to university. Although it may not be your first choice of course or university, there are degrees available to those with Australian Tertiary Admission Rank (ATAR) scores of 50.00 and above. As long as you have marks sufficient to get you into *any* undergraduate degree at an Australian university, you have the chance to sit the GAMSAT and apply for graduate medicine. If you don't get into university straight out of high school, there are other ways to get into university. These include studying at TAFE which will then allow you to enter university, and try to get into graduate medicine. In fact, most people enter their medical degrees as graduates for a range of different reasons.

The benefits of undergraduate medicine include:

- You finish your degree and training at a younger age, so are not studying in a training program while you are of the age to start a family – and so undergraduate degrees are said to be more family and female friendly.
- The degree is longer (between 5 and 6 years in duration) allowing more time to balance your learning and other interests.
- You will be employed at a similar age to others of your age group (as opposed to graduate medicine, where you may start work years after people you went to high school with).

The benefits of graduate medicine include:

- Increased maturity and prior work experience.
- The degree is shorter (usually 4 years in duration).

Undergraduate Medical School Application Timeline

A timeline of the undergraduate medical school application, along with recommendations on when to start preparing is shown below:

<u>Final year of high school:</u>

January:	Start studying for the UMAT and consider completing extra-curricular activities.
April:	UMAT registrations open. Begin preparing your application.
May – September:	Applications to individual universities close (check with your preferred medical school for specific dates).
June:	UMAT registrations close.
July:	UMAT exam.
September:	UMAT results are released.
October – November:	Sit higher school certificate.
November – January:	Offers for interview are sent. Start preparing for your interview now!
January:	Interviews are held.
January – February:	Medical school offers are sent.
Late February – March:	Undergraduate medical degrees commence.

Graduate Medical School Application Timeline

A timeline of the graduate medical school application, along with recommendations on when to start preparing for each step is shown below:

October the previous year: GAMSAT registrations open.

November the previous year: Start studying for the GAMSAT.

January: GAMSAT registrations close.

March: GAMSAT exam.

May: GAMSAT results are available. Start preparing your application.

May – June: Applications to medical schools are due.

June: Offers for interview are sent. Start preparing for the interview.

July – October: Interviews are held.

September – November: Medical school offers are sent.

February the next year: Graduate medical schools commence.

5 | Undergraduate Entry into Medical School and the UMAT

1) *Decide medicine is for you*

2) ***Position yourself:***

    a. ***Optimise marks in high school or university***

    b. ***Obtain extra-curricular experience***

3) ***Study and sit for the entry exams (UMAT or GAMSAT)***

4) *Prepare and submit your application*

5) *Prepare for and sit your interview*

6) *Accept your invitation to medical school*

Universities that Offer Undergraduate Medicine

As a school leaver, you have many choices of universities for medical school (and not just within Australia – one university in New Zealand offers medicine to Australian citizens). These are categorised by state, and include:

- New South Wales:
  - University of New South Wales
  - University of Newcastle/University of New England (Joint Medical Program)
  - University of Western Sydney
- Victoria:
  - Monash University
- South Australia:
  - University of Adelaide
  - Flinders University

- Queensland:
  - Bond University
  - James Cook University
  - University of Queensland (Provisional Entry)*
- Tasmania:
  - University of Tasmania
- Western Australia:
  - University of Western Australia (Provisional Entry)*
- New Zealand:
  - University of Otago

Provisional entry means that you can be admitted into a program where you complete an under-graduate degree (such as a Bachelor of Medical Science), before you begin your graduate medical degree. This way, you don't have to sit the GAMSAT to get into a graduate medical degree – and would graduate with a Bachelor of Science, as well as a medical degree.

General Undergraduate Entry Requirements

As outlined in Chapter 2: 'Characteristics of Doctor', there are several characteristics sought by the selection panel of the aforementioned universities for undergraduate entry into medicine. In no particular order, these include academic ability, empathy, communication, teamwork and leadership. Four criteria are used to assess how applicants perform on the above characteristics:

- High school marks (ATAR/TER/ENTER/OP) – assesses the academic standing of applicants
- Application – assesses the teamwork and leadership skills of applicants
- UMAT score – assesses the academic level and empathic skills of applicants
- Interview[†] – assesses the communication, empathic, teamwork and leadership skills of applicants (See Chapter 9: 'The Interview')

[†] *University of Tasmania no longer interviews applicants for their medical program.*

Keep in mind that extra-curricular activities are highly regarded in both the application and the interview. Thus, ensure you have carried out activities such as those mentioned in Chapter 8: 'The Application'.

Each university has different entry requirements, with different scores required for admission (see Chapter 12: 'University Information').

High School Marks and Subjects

There is a high demand for entry into undergraduate medicine, and as such it means universities can often select only those who score in the 95th percentile or above. It is best to establish a good routine and effective study techniques early in high school. The last few years of high school (Years 10–12) are the most important, so ensure you have already learnt how to optimise your study techniques prior to this (see Chapter 3: 'Study Techniques'). There is such a thing as working too hard for too long, however, and 'burn out' is something to be avoided, or you won't be able to maximise your marks.

It is important to note that most medical schools have high school subjects as prerequisites. That is, many medical schools require you to have studied English, maths, biology and/or chemistry, and some may require other subjects. Contact your preferred medical school to find out what high school subjects they require you to have completed (*contact details of each medical school are found in Chapter 12*). Keep in mind summer schools are available if you have not completed these prerequisite subjects prior to university. However if you have the option to complete these subjects at school you will be ahead of those trying to do a quick catch up course at summer school.

> *'Choose subjects that you enjoy, and don't worry too much about scaling. The two subjects I did that I felt helped me most at uni were biology and PDHPE, which are both apparently 'low scaling' – but I loved them so I did well in them, and that basic knowledge was really useful as a transition point in first year uni.'*
>
> Anika Johnston, High Distinction Student, Sixth Year Medicine, University of New South Wales

UMAT

Introduction to the UMAT

The Undergraduate Medicine and Health Sciences Admission Test or UMAT (www.umat.acer.edu.au), was first implemented at the University of Newcastle over twenty years ago, and has spread throughout Australia as part of the medical and dental selection process. It is an aptitude test designed to assess a student's logical, reasoning, empathic and problem solving skills. The UMAT consists of 122 multiple choice questions (with 4 options, A through D) to be answered within 2 hours and 45 minutes of test time. It is run by the Australian Council for Educational Research (ACER) and is generally held in late July. Like all medical entry tests it is supposed to be impossible to prepare for (and in fact, the UMAT website states that 'intensive preparation is not advisable or necessary'), but you certainly *can* get better at answering these types of questions if you practice, and thus improve your chance of doing well.

Anyone who is in their last year of high school (or has already completed high school) can sit the UMAT. Registrations open early April, and close late May or early June (in 2012, registrations closed on 1 June). You must register online at www. umat.acer.edu.au. The exam itself is held in late July (in 2012 it was held on 25 July), and results take around two months to become available – in 2012, results were emailed out in late September. Results will be given as a score for each section of the test, your overall score and your overall percentile rank (how you compared to others). Sitting the UMAT costs $200, with additional fees if registration is late or if you wish to sit the UMAT outside Australia or New Zealand.

There are numerous sites in each state which offer the UMAT, and even some overseas. These include:

- New South Wales:
  - Armidale
  - Dubbo
  - Newcastle
  - Sydney
- Victoria:
  - Bendigo
  - Geelong
  - Melbourne
  - Mildura
  - Sale
  - Shepparton
- Australian Capital Territory:
  - Canberra
- Northern Territory:
  - Alice Springs
  - Darwin
- Queensland:
  - Brisbane
  - Cairns
  - Gold Coast
  - Townsville
- South Australia:
  - Adelaide
- Western Australia:
  - Perth
- New Zealand:
  - Auckland
  - Dunedin
- Singapore
- United Kingdom:
  - London
- United States:
  - Washington DC

Sections of the UMAT

Although the test itself takes 2 hours and 45 minutes, the whole process will take you between 4 and 6 hours, including reporting to the testing centre and breaks between parts of the exam. The best way to study for the UMAT is to complete UMAT-specific questions like those below (see Appendix A for more practice UMAT questions). The UMAT comprises 3 sections:

Section 1 – Logical Reasoning and Problem Solving (65 minutes)

This section consists of 44 questions. A piece of information (in the format of either a block of text or a graph) is given and requires you to use logic and reasoning to deduce the answer from the presented stimulus. This section seeks to examine the language capabilities of the student, so while the content is not necessarily technical, it does require a fairly advanced level of comprehension. The stimulus may or may not be of a scientific/medical nature, and can come from any source.

Example: A study is trialling a new drug for migraine headaches, and comparing its effect to an old anti-migraine drug. The trial has 4 groups of 250 people each: Group 1 is given nothing, Group 2 is given the old drug (Migrainex), Group 3 is given the new drug (Migraine-ease) and Group 4 is given a sugar pill with no active ingredients (placebo). The patients in Group 1 do not improve at all, patients in Group 2 improved by 30 percent, patients in Group 3 improved by 60 percent, and patients in Group 4 improved by 30 percent. Choose the correct statement:

A) All groups had an equal improvement

B) All drugs were equally effective

C) Migrainex was twice as effective as Migraine-ease

D) Some patients improved even though they weren't given any real anti-migraine medication

D is the correct answer. They will often make you reach the next level of reasoning in your answer. For example, they won't just say 'Migrainex had no better effect than the placebo' (which is true), but will make you reach the conclusion that follows this ('Some patients improved even though they weren't given any real anti-migraine medication'). Keep in mind, they will often give you extra information (for example, that there were 250 people in each group, or the names of the drugs) to distract you.

Section 2 – Understanding People (50 minutes)

This consists of 40 questions. This section tests how you respond to situations involving other people, mainly assessing your level of empathy. A scenario is presented, and you are asked to infer the feelings, thoughts, intentions and possible responses of the people in the scenario.

Example: A couple (Person A and Person B) are served the wrong food in a restaurant. Person A is allergic to nuts, and is served a dish that may contain peanuts. How are they most likely to feel?

A) Person A – depressed and moody; Person B – happy and unconcerned

B) Person A – frightened and anxious; Person B – irritated and concerned for his/her partner

C) Person A – appreciative; Person B – angry and frustrated

D) Person A – happy and unconcerned; Person B – sad and fearful

B is the correct answer, as Person A (who has a nut allergy) is likely to be anxious and frightened about the near miss, while Person B is likely to be very worried about the health of his/her partner. As mentioned earlier, empathy is the ability to guess what other people are thinking, so try putting yourself in the shoes of the people in the scenarios.

Section 3 – Non-verbal Reasoning (50 minutes)

This section consists of 38 questions, and assesses your non-verbal reasoning by presenting you with a sequence of shapes and asking you to guess what the next shape should be, given the pattern.

Example: Which pattern should follow? Choose from the options below (A–D):

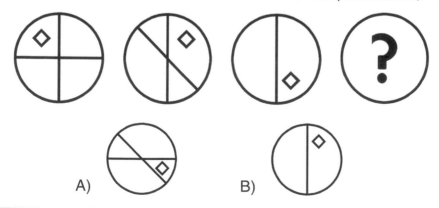

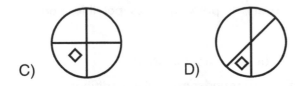

C)   D)

The correct answer is D. This section often overwhelms people, but you can answer these if you have a system. Address the problem one part at a time. In the example, notice how the diamond is moving clockwise, one quarter at a time – therefore, in the fourth shape, it will be in the bottom left corner. Next, look at the lines. Note how the vertical line remains still, but the other line moves clockwise by 45° each time (so although it looks like it disappears in the third shape, it is really just hidden by the stationary vertical line) – therefore the fourth shape will have the vertical line still as always, and the moving line rotated clockwise an extra 45°.

How to Study for the UMAT

The UMAT body advises not to spend hours and hours practicing UMAT-type questions. This is good advice, as you should simultaneously be studying to optimise your high school marks. However, like anything in life, practice does help, and so you should spend some time getting used to UMAT-style questions and conditions.

The UMAT body produces two booklets which each contain a full-length practice UMAT exam. These booklets will give you an idea of the type of questions, the content, and the timing expected. Use these booklets to identify your strengths and weaknesses, so you can target your study to focus on your weaker areas. For other useful resources see the 'UMAT, GAMSAT and Study Techniques' section in the back of the book.

> *'You can memorise anything as long as you repeat it often enough.'*
>
> Associate Professor Nigel Hope, Consultant Orthopaedic Surgeon, Sydney Adventist Hospital

Once you are within a couple of weeks of the UMAT, I would recommend sitting down and undergoing the practice tests. Find a quiet spot with no distractions, set a stopwatch and adhere to the exact timing of the UMAT test. This will give you an idea how you need to pace yourself during the exam, the stress of the exam, and will give you a last chance to work out if you have any weak areas.

To give yourself as much preparation as possible, consider doing the following:

- Complete practice questions for the UMAT
- Complete practice exams under exam-like conditions
- Consider completing a preparation course (see below)

Q: What is your favourite part of medical school?

A: *My cohort. I have really enjoyed forming some solid relationships with my peers and I anticipate that many will remain friends for life.*

Dr Ed Campion, Intern, St Vincent's Hospital, Sydney

Useful Resources

For the UMAT you can buy similar books to those booklets provided by the UMAT body from your local book shop or online (e.g. through Amazon) that will test your comprehension (Section 1), your ability to solve puzzles (Section 3) and possibly even your ability to understand people (Section 2) (see the Further Reading section for books to better your UMAT skills). In addition you can purchase UMAT textbooks from ACER (see the UMAT website at www.umat.acer.edu.au).

Another good source of UMAT practice materials is from older students, especially those that are already studying medicine. However, it is often 'first in best dressed', so once you decide to sit the UMAT, ask these people as soon as possible, before other people do!

The Medical College Admissions Test (MCAT) is the test used in the United States to select medical applicants, and is similar to the UMAT and GAMSAT. There are plenty of sources willing to sell MCAT questions, which is another good source of practice materials which can be purchased online. Similarly, the Graduate Management Admissions Test (GMAT) is a test used in the United States to select for applicants into graduate business programs, with some sections similar to the UMAT and GAMSAT (while some are quite different) – this is another source of practice questions that you can purchase online. Just search Amazon and you will find many books of practice questions.

Preparation Courses for the UMAT

The UMAT body (the Australian Council for Educational Research – ACER) does not recommend any specific preparation courses, and in fact says that 'some commercial preparation courses might provide misleading information or advice to candidates'. Preparation courses often charge large fees and pretend that they have 'secrets' on the UMAT that will help get you great marks. Although they are often extremely expensive (sometimes over $1,000), any practice is helpful, so you may want to consider one of these courses. With this in mind, many people do not do these courses and are still successful in gaining entry into medical school.

The Day before the UMAT

A few tips:

- Try to limit your study the day before the exam. You will perform better if you are rested and relaxed.
- Ensure that you have the equipment required for the UMAT.
- Set an alarm for the morning (and ask a family member or friend to set theirs too), giving yourself adequate time.
- Go to bed early and avoid alcohol, coffee or anything which will keep you awake or interfere with your sleep.

Things you MUST bring to the UMAT:

- Your UMAT admission ticket (which is sent to you upon registering for the UMAT)
- Photo identification (current drivers license, passport, or proof of age card)
- Lead pencils (at least 3, because once the test has started you don't want to be sharpening broken or blunt pencils, or trying to borrow them from the examiners), preferably Medium–Soft Number 2 or HB
- An eraser
- A watch to monitor your timing

There is often nowhere to store personal items at the examination site, and as such I would recommend you bring as little as possible. Consider bringing a bottle of water as it is a long test and you don't want to get dehydrated.

On the Day of the UMAT

A few tips:

- Give yourself adequate time to get ready and to get to the examination site.
- Have a low glycaemic index breakfast (e.g., cereal, toast) to keep your energy levels up throughout the day.

- Double check that you have all the required equipment with you (i.e., admission ticket, identification, pencils etc. See above).

- Pack yourself lunch and snacks or bring money to buy food.

- Arrive to the examination site early, and use take this time to relax before the examination.

- All of the questions in the UMAT are multiple choice and they all have the same value – so there is no point in answering some questions and not others. You improve your chances if you answer as many questions as possible, leaving none out – even if this means you have to guess a few towards the end if you are running out of time. Marks are not deducted for wrong answers – so answer every question.

- Answer every question from start to finish.

- If you have difficulty with a question, mark that question in your question book and come back to it at the end.

- Don't spend too long on any particular question – rather move on and answer more questions before you run out of time.

- Choose your answer by the process of elimination. Cross out those answers that you know are wrong and then you can begin to deduce which answer is most likely right. Even if you have to guess between the last two, you have improved your chances from 25 percent to 50 percent.

- Circle your answers on the question sheet as a draft, but don't forget to transcribe your answers onto your answer sheet straight away – do not leave this until the end!

Time is limited in the UMAT which helps to separate those students that work well under a time pressure. If you want to be a doctor, you must have the ability to work under these conditions, so just remind yourself of that.

UMAT examiners take the exam very seriously, and you can be disqualified from the test (and possibly from sitting the UMAT in the future) if you are seen carrying:

- Stationery apart from a pencil and eraser
- Mobile phones
- Calculators
- Stopwatches

- Dictionaries
- Recording devices
- Food (unless you have a medical certificate indicating you need it for medical reasons)
- Bags

Further, you can suffer similar penalties if you lie during the registration process, copy any part of the test to take with you upon leaving, work on a part of the exam you have not yet been instructed to work on, or give or receive assistance to or from others.

Now you have prepared for this test for months, so do not stress! You have put in the hard work, and it is about to pay off. Just keep calm, answer everything you can and you will surprise yourself.

Good luck!

6 | Graduate Entry into Medical School and the GAMSAT

1) *Decide medicine is for you*

2) ***Position yourself:***

    a. ***Optimise marks in high school or university***

    b. ***Obtain extra-curricular experience***

3) ***Study and sit for the entry exams (UMAT or GAMSAT)***

4) *Prepare and submit your application*

5) *Prepare for and sit your interview*

6) *Accept your invitation to medical school*

Universities that Offer Graduate Medicine

As a graduate, you have many choices of universities for medical school, which include:

- New South Wales:
  - University of Sydney
  - University of Notre Dame (Sydney)
  - University of Wollongong
- Victoria:
  - University of Melbourne
  - Monash University
  - Deakin University

- South Australia:
  - Flinders University
- Queensland:
  - University of Queensland
  - Griffith University
- Western Australia:
  - University of Western Australia
  - University of Notre Dame (Fremantle)
- Australian Capital Territory:
  - Australian National University
- New Zealand
  - University of Otago

General Graduate Entry Requirements

As discussed in the undergraduate chapter, there are several characteristics sought by the selection panel of graduate medical schools. Three criteria[*] are used to assess how applicants perform on the characteristics of empathy, academic ability, communication, teamwork and leadership:

- University marks (using the Grade Point Average, or GPA)
- GAMSAT score
- Interview[†]

[*] *Some universities, such as the University of Notre Dame and the University of Wollongong require applicants to submit a supplementary form, where you list your achievements, goals and why you wish to study at that particular university. This is dealt with more in Chapter 8: 'The Application'.*

[†] *Some universities (including the University of Queensland) no longer interview applicants for the graduate program.*

Keep in mind that extra-curricular activities are highly regarded in both the application and the interview. Thus, ensure you have carried out activities such as those mentioned in Chapter 8: 'The Application'.

Each medical school has different requirements for each of these criteria. The GPA and GAMSAT scores required are listed in Chapter 12: 'University Information' with information on the individual universities.

University Marks

University marks are used to screen for potential applicants, so you will not be offered an interview if your GPA (Grade Point Average, which is a way of measuring your university marks that is slightly different to an average of your percentages for each subject) is not high enough.

GPA calculations differ slightly at each university, but generally the equivalent percentage to GPA is as follows:

• 50–64% equates to a GPA of 4.5

• 65–74% equates to a GPA of 5.75

• 75–84% equates to a GPA of 6.75

• 85% and above equates to a GPA of 7

Different universities have different cut-off GPA marks (below which you will not get an interview – see the entry requirements for each medical school in Chapter 12: 'University Information'). The higher your GPA is above the cut off, the greater your chance of getting an offer to medical school. See Chapter 3: 'Study Techniques' for tips on how to optimise your study techniques and achieve the highest marks you can.

Some graduate medical schools weight the GPAs, with the first year of the undergraduate degree multiplied by 1, the second year multiplied by 2 and the third year multiplied by 3 (so the later years are weighted more heavily). Contact your chosen medical school for more information (see Chapter 12: 'University Information' for information on the individual medical schools).

GAMSAT

Introduction to the GAMSAT

The Graduate Australian Medical School Admissions Test or GAMSAT (www.gamsat-ie.org/gamsat-australia) is used throughout Australia for selecting medical school applicants who have already completed a tertiary degree (a degree at university). Similar to the UMAT, it is a test which assesses academic ability, although unlike the UMAT, it focuses on 'high level intellectual studies', namely basic concepts of science, problem solving, critical thinking and writing, and the ability to apply these in different situations.

The GAMSAT comprises 3 sections, consisting of 185 multiple choice questions (of which there are 4 options, A through D) and two short essays, to be completed in five and a half hours (with a one hour break between Section 2 and Section 3). It is run by ACER (the Australian Council for Educational Research) and is generally held in mid to late March. Preparation is a must for the GAMSAT, as it is essential that you know your physics, chemistry, biology, essay writing, comprehension and critical analysis. Also, just like the UMAT, practicing the types of questions asked will improve your chances of doing well.

'I love that the body becomes a complex puzzle, and the challenge is figuring out which piece of the puzzle has gone wrong. I also find it very humbling that a complete stranger puts so much trust in a doctor (or even medical student) that they let you know the intimate and private details of their life, simply so they can improve their health.'

Emily Sutherland, High Distinction Student, Sixth Year Medicine, University of New South Wales

Anyone who is in their second-last or last year of a 3 year (or greater length) degree can sit the GAMSAT. If you have completed a degree within the last 10 years, you may sit the GAMSAT – but if you completed your degree over 10 years ago, contact your specific medical school to check your eligibility.

You can use your GAMSAT mark for 2 years after you have sat it. A technique many people use is to sit the GAMSAT in their second last year of university, and again in their last year. This way, you see what the test is like (as well as having covered the basic sciences in the first year of your science degree, or having just learnt how to write essays and critically analyse text in the first year of your arts degree), and if your mark is not outstanding you can sit the GAMSAT again in your final year – but this time, you know what you are expecting!

Registrations for GAMSAT open in the previous October and close late January or early February (in 2012, registrations closed on the first of February), and are completed online – see the above address. The GAMSAT is held in late March (in 2012, it was held on 24 March), with results available mid-May. Your results will be given as a score for each of the 3 sections, as well as an overall GAMSAT score – these are given on a scale of 0 to 100, but they are not percentage marks (no one apart from the ACER people are sure why they score it this way). The overall GAMSAT score is calculated as [(Section 1 + Section 2 + 2 × Section 3) divided by 4], so as you can see Section 3 (the science section) is weighted more heavily than the rest (although Melbourne University does not weight the GAMSAT this way). The cost of sitting the GAMSAT is $409, with additional fees if you wish to sit the exam overseas – although this does include a booklet of sample questions.

There are numerous sites in each state which offer the GAMSAT, and even some overseas.

These include:

- New South Wales:
  - Sydney
- Victoria:
  - Melbourne
- Australian Capital Territory:
  - Canberra
- Northern Territory:
  - Darwin
- Queensland:
  - Brisbane
  - Townsville
- South Australia:
  - Adelaide
- Western Australia:
  - Perth
- New Zealand:
  - Wellington
- Singapore
- United Kingdom:
  - London
- United States:
  - Washington DC

Note that the United Kingdom GAMSAT is held in September (in 2012 was on the 21 September) and they have a testing centre in Melbourne, Australia. This costs £100 in addition to the usual registration fee (not including the cost of flights and accommodation in Melbourne!). The UK GAMSAT is directly comparable to the Australian GAMSAT, and marks are accepted by some Australian universities (contact your preferred medical school for more information). However, as it is held in September it is too late in the year to allow admission the following year. Therefore, the September UK GAMSAT can be used for entry in two years' time, or can be used as practice for an attempt at the Australian GAMSAT the following year.

Sections of the GAMSAT

The GAMSAT comprises 3 sections:

Section 1 – Reasoning in Humanities and Social Sciences (100 minutes)

This section consists of 75 multiple choice (with 4 options, A through D) comprehension and critical analysis questions. Section 1 assesses your understanding and interpretation of non-science writing such as poetry, essays, newspaper articles and some images and tables. There are 3 main types of question: understanding explicit and implicit meanings in text and images, reasoning and drawing conclusions, and critical thinking. Generally, you will be presented with a large block of text from which they will ask you several questions, testing your comprehension and understanding, asking you to draw a conclusion from the information given, or asking you to criticise the writer. The text may be taken from poetry, novels, newspapers or textbooks to give you variety and make sure you can interpret information from various sources.

Example:

> *'Stand you awhile apart, Confine yourself but in a patient list.*
> *Whilst you were here o'erwhelmèd with your grief—*
> *A passion most resulting such a man—*
> *Cassio came hither. I shifted him away*
> *And laid good 'scuses upon your ecstasy…'*
> From Shakespeare's *Othello*

What is the speaker most likely trying to say?

A) 'Go somewhere else and calm down. I made an excuse to Cassio about your grief, which, by the way, doesn't suit you.'

B) 'Stand separately, be patient, and put yourself on the waiting list. While you were grieving, the passionate Cassio came, but I made him wait too.'

C) 'Stand apart and confine yourself. Your grief is a passion resulting from the man Cassio, whom I distracted.'

D) 'Keep to yourself and be patient. Cassio came while you were overwhelmed with grief – an emotion that becomes you – but I asked him to leave.'

The correct answer is A. I found this the most difficult section, and while not all of the questions are from poetry (which often relies on interpretation), some are. If you struggled with this question, I would recommend getting a book on interpreting poetry, or visiting www.sparknotes.com.

Section 2 – Written Communication (60 minutes)

In this section you are required to write two essays in response to one of a handful of related quotes (for example, you may be able to choose between 5 quotes on imagination, two of which may be: 'Imagination is more important than knowledge' (Albert Einstein), and 'He who has imagination without learning, has wings and no feet' (Joseph Joubert). It is essential that you address both sides of the argument, instead of just agreeing with the quote – that is, instead of agreeing with Einstein that imagination *is* more important than knowledge, you also should argue the opposite case, giving evidence that knowledge may sometimes be more important than imagination. This shows that you have an open mind and can see multiple views of a topic, and can discuss these openly. It is also helpful to give examples, to bolster your arguments. Assessors will consider what is said (the quality of the ideas, and how well it is argued), as well as how it is said (including introductory and concluding sentences or paragraphs, sentence structure, and grammar). Ensure you choose the quote which you find easiest to write about.

Example:

'The future depends on what we do in the present'
Mahatma Gandhi

Section 3 – Reasoning in Biological and Physical Sciences (170 minutes)

This section consists of 110 multiple choice science questions (with four options, A through D). As mentioned above, this section assesses your ability to recall and utilise concepts in the sciences. They will be testing Year 11 and Year 12 physics, and first year university chemistry and biology (including organic chemistry). See below for a detailed list of topics to cover in each of these areas. In this section they are looking for applicants to be able to understand and apply scientific concepts, make generalisations, interpret data, translate knowledge from one format to another, make comparisons, apply hypotheses, evaluate the quality of the evidence, extrapolate and interpolate. While this sounds complex, it is nothing you haven't already encountered in your science degree – or if you come from a non-science background, can't pick up when studying science textbooks before the exam. The data will be provided as text, graphs, images, tables and diagrams. For example, the chemistry questions may be posed as drawings of molecules that are to interact, ball and stick drawings for organic chemistry, or simple chemical equations. In Section 3, 40 percent of the questions are on chemistry, 40 percent on biology and 20 percent on physics. As mentioned above, the science section is weighted more heavily than the other sections so it is essential that you have a thorough knowledge of the sciences and perform as well as possible on Section 3.

Example: The thyroid gland is a bi-lobed gland located in the neck. It takes iodine from the body and converts it into the thyroid hormones triiodothyronine (T3) and thyroxine (T4), which regulate the metabolic rate of the body. The release of T3 and T4 is under the control of the hypothalamus, via a negative-feedback loop. The hypothalamus senses the amount of T3 and T4 in the blood, so when levels of T3 and T4 drop, the hypothalamus releases Thyrotropin-Releasing Hormone (TRH). This TRH acts on the pituitary gland to cause release of Thyroid Stimulating Hormone (TSH). The TSH then diffuses to the thyroid gland, which it stimulates to release T3 and T4. Once enough T3 and T4 are released, the hypothalamus decreases the amount of TRH released, so a balance is reached.

What would happen if the thyroid became insensitive to TSH?

A) Levels of T3 would increase, while T4 would decrease

B) The production of thyroid hormones would decrease

C) Levels of TSH would decrease

D) Levels of TRH would decrease

The correct answer is B, as TSH is the stimulus that causes release of the thyroid hormones (T3 and T4), and if the thyroid gland is not responding to TSH, then T3 and T4 will not be produced by the thyroid. It may be easier if you quickly sketch a diagram showing the flow of events, which may look something like:

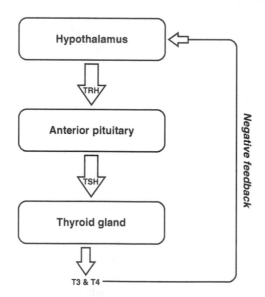

How and What to Study for the GAMSAT

It is important to optimise your university marks whilst studying for the GAMSAT. Your university marks are used in the selection process so you want to ensure that these are outstanding whilst still being prepared for the GAMSAT.

Many applicants complete a Bachelor of Science degree at university in preparation for the GAMSAT. A science degree will cover chemistry, biology and occasionally physics, which will be required for Section 3 of the GAMSAT. However, these science subjects can also be learnt over a few months through self study, and as such many applicants complete other degrees (arts, architecture, finance and other non-science degrees). Non-science degrees can also offer advantages to applicants such as those in which there is a greater focus on essay writing, comprehension and critical thinking.

As the exam is held in mid- to late March, I recommended that you start studying for the GAMSAT in the November of the previous year, when the university semester ends (refer to the timeline of the process in Chapter 4). This gives you approximately 3 months to prepare. I recommend that you set up a calendar or timetable (see Chapter 5: 'Study Techniques'), plan out the topics within each subject that you will need to cover and allocate these to your calendar. I recommend that you aim to finish your study by the end of January, and allocate practice questions and papers to February.

The GAMSAT body produces two booklets which each contain a half-length practice GAMSAT exam, and a booklet of sample questions which come free with your GAMSAT registration. I found it useful to flick through the book of sample questions to indicate the type of questions and the timing required, before looking at anything else. This helped me work out what was expected – as well as my strengths and weaknesses – indicating where I should be focussing my study time. Practice questions for the GAMSAT can be found in Appendix B.

Tips on How to Prepare for the GAMSAT

- Purchase the university prescribed textbooks for the subjects you are required to cover (i.e., physics, chemistry, biology), as well as books on essay writing and comprehension.

- Start from the beginning of the book (i.e., the introduction) and make your way through the book, building on the basics. Don't skip chapters as you will need to be building on the basic knowledge and if you lack this you will end up having to go back and relearn those topics.

- Make notes on each chapter/topic as you go (refer to study tips) which can then be used to review if needed later on.

- Practice your essay writing and comprehension skills.

- Complete a preparation course (see below).

- Complete practice questions and do so under a time constraint.

> **Q:** What was your favourite part of medical school?
>
> **A:** *Excellent teachers whose lectures I still remember twenty-five years on.*
>
> Dr Elspeth Fotheringham, General Practitioner, Tuggerah

What to Study for the GAMSAT

Below are tips and recommendations on what to study for the sections relating to comprehension, essays, physics, biology, chemistry, organic chemistry and mathematics.

<u>Comprehension</u>: For both Sections 1 and 3, the stimulus material may be a simple graph, but it is often a dense half-page block of text, or several complex graphs or pieces of data to be considered together. As such, it is essential to read quickly through the material while processing and understanding it. Reading quickly and effectively may not be a skill you already have, but practice can improve this. Prepare for this section by finding large blocks of text and complex graphs (for example from newspapers and textbooks), and working on finding a balance between reading through them as fast as possible, while progressing slowly enough to understand the content. After a bit of practice in doing this, you will find yourself speeding up considerably while retaining much of what you have read. Something I found especially useful were GMAT practice tests, which have many questions similar to Section 1 of the GAMSAT. You can buy GMAT question books online at the GMAT website (www.mba.com/the-gmat.aspx) or via Amazon.

<u>Essays</u>: I am sure you can find hundreds of good books on writing great essays, and I recommend you work your way through at least one of these. Find quotes like the ones given in the examples (and in Appendix B), and practice writing an essay with an introductory sentence, arguments for and against the quote and a concluding sentence, all within 30 minutes, and then have a family member or friend mark them. I guarantee you get better with practice! Another great technique is to get one of the short essay books written by philosopher A. C. Grayling (see the References section for some of his books). He takes a quote, much like the ones you will be given, and writes a short essay with great arguments and counter arguments, which is written exactly as you should be writing yours (although his may be slightly longer).

<u>Physics</u>: Topics recommended to cover:

• The definition of dependent variables, independent variables and controls

- *Electricity and the electromagnetic spectrum*: waves (including wavelength, frequency, velocity, amplitude, displacement, pitch, crests, troughs, superposition), types of radiation in the electromagnetic spectrum, absorption, reflection and refraction of light, mirrors, lenses, the inverse square law, Snell's law, voltage, resistance and current, parallel and series circuits, electric fields (including field strength, force, charge), conductors and insulators, generators, potential differences, magnets (including magnetic fields, the right-hand grip rule, magnetic flux, Lenz's Law).

- *Movement*: force, mass and acceleration, distance, speed and time, Newton's laws, scalar and vector quantities, velocities, acceleration, gravity and gravitational fields, conservation of energy, centripetal forces, momentum, projectile motion, friction, inclined planes, collisions, torque, kinetic and potential energy.

Recommended topics come from the HSC Physics Syllabus, at www.boardof studies.nsw.edu.au/syllabus_hsc/physics.html

Biology: Topics recommended to cover:

- Cell biology (especially how cells obtain and use energy, osmosis, and so on).

- Molecular biology (including DNA and protein synthesis).

- Genetics.

- Current technology for DNA analysis.

- Theories of evolution.

Suggested topics for biology study were taken from the Biology Course Outline at the University of Sydney website at http://sydney.edu.au/courses/uos/BIOL1001/ concepts-in-biology

Chemistry: Topics recommended to cover:

- *Elements and atoms*: elements, compounds and mixtures, physical and chemical change, chemical symbols, atomic structure, protons, electrons, neutrons, atomic number, isotopes, radioactivity, shell structure.

- *Molecules and ions*: formation of ions, ionic compound formation, formulas and naming, covalent bonding, valence, and bonding and non-bonding pairs, double and triple bonds, naming covalent compounds, polyatomic ions, empirical, molecular and structural formulas, types of bonding in solids.

- *Chemical equations*: reaction types (combination, precipitation, decomposition, replacement, acid/base), molecular/ionic equations, specification of phase, balancing equations for neutral and charged species, reactions involving acids.

- *Stoichiometry*: atomic, formula and molecular weights, the Avogadro constant, the mole and molar mass, percent composition, empirical and molecular formulas, calculations involving balanced equations, limiting reagents and percentage yield, molarity and calculations on solutions.

- *The periodic table.*

- *Atomic energy levels*: shapes of atomic orbitals and quantum numbers.

- *The Lewis model of bonding*: Lewis structure, pi bonding, resonance.

- *VSEPR*: molecular shape, application to larger molecules including organic molecules, shape and bonding of common functional groups.

- *Liquid crystals*: packing determined by shape.

- *Gas laws*: effects of temperature and pressure on volume, the ideal gas law.

- *Thermochemistry*: heat and temperature, kinetic and potential energy, the First Law of Thermodynamics, heat capacity, enthalpy and endo- and exothermic reactions, Hess's Law, heat of formation, energy release from fuels.

- *Types of intermolecular forces*: dipole, induced dipole, dispersion and hydrogen bonding, effects on boiling points.

- *Oxidation numbers.*

- *Chemical equilibrium*: equilibrium as a dynamic process, the equilibrium constant, the reaction quotient, predicting direction of chemical change, equilibrium calculations, Kp and partial pressures, Kc and units of concentration, Ksp, equilibrium calculations, Ka and Kb, pKa and pKb, Le Chatelier's principle.

- *Electrochemistry*: oxidation states, redox reactions, cell potential, half-reactions, voltaic cells, galvanic cells, the Nernst equation, the link between E and K.

Organic chemistry: Topics recommended to cover:

- *Molecular structure*: bonding and shape, shape and hybridisation for alkanes, alkenes and alkynes, stick notation, functional groups and nomenclature.

- *Alkanes*: constitutional isomers, conformational isomers, cis/trans isomers of cyclic alkanes.

- *Alkenes*: pi-bonds and structure, E/Z isomers, introduction to organic mechanisms, addition reactions, mechanism of electrophilic addition, Markovnikov's rule.

- *Aromatic compounds*.

- *Alcohols*: structure of alcohols, phenols and ethers, H-bonding and physical properties of alcohols, acid–base reactions of alcohols and phenols, oxidation reactions, elimination reactions and Zaitsev's rule.

- *Amines*: structure of amines, H-bonding and physical properties of amines, amines as bases,

- *Stereochemistry*: stereogenic centres, optical activity, (R) and (S) nomenclature, racemic mixtures, chirality.

- *Organic halogen compounds*: substitiution reactions, SN2 mechanism, elimination reactions.

- *Aldehydes and ketones*: structure and polarity, nucleophilic addition reactions of hydride reducing agents, oxidation of aldehydes.

- *Carboxylic acids and derivatives*: carboxylic acids, acidity and resonance stabilisation of conjugate bases, reduction to primary alcohols, formation of acid chlorides, derivatives (acid halides, anhydrides, esters and amides, acid halides, anhydrides, esters and amides, relative reactivity of carboxylic acid derivatives, interconversion and hydrolysis of derivatives, polymers.

- *Strong acids and bases*: electrolytes, autoionisation of water, conjugate acid–base pairs.

- *Weak acids and bases*: carboxylic acids, carbonic acids, phenols, ammonia, amines.

- *Calculations involving pKa and pKb*: buffers, the common ion effect.

- *Intermolecular forces and phase behaviour*: boiling point trends, solid structure (ice, etc.).

- *Solubility equilibrium*: calculations involving Ksp, solubility trends as a function of polarity of solvents (e.g., alcohols in water), solubility of ionic solids, role of intermolecular forces in solubility, heats of salvation.

- *Kinetics*: variability of reaction rates, review of first order rate constants and radioactive decay, mechanism and rate determining steps, temperature and the Arrhenius relation, catalysis, enzymes.

Suggestions of material to cover for chemistry came from the Sydney University School of Chemistry Website, at http://firstyear.chem.usyd.edu.au/chem1001/ *and* http://firstyear.chem.usyd.edu.au/chem1002/.

<u>Maths</u>: While not a distinct category for assessment, you cannot hope to pass the science section without a good understanding of mathematics. This is especially true as no calculators are allowed in the exam, so make sure you can multiply and divide large numbers (for example, (6×10^9) times (5×10^8). If you have problems completing practice questions while studying for chemistry, physics and biology, consider revising basic mathematics.

Useful Resources

For the GAMSAT you can buy similar books to the booklets provided by the GAMSAT body from your local book shop or online (e.g., through Amazon). In addition, look in the chapters of any physics, chemistry and biology textbooks for practice questions for Section 3. In addition you can purchase GAMSAT textbooks from ACER (see the GAMSAT website at www.gamsat-ie.org/gamsat-australia).

Another good source of GAMSAT practice materials is from older students, especially those that are already studying medicine. However, it is often 'first in best dressed', so once you decide to sit the GAMSAT, ask these people as soon as possible, before other people do!

The Medical College Admissions Test (MCAT) is the test used in the United States to select medical applicants, and is similar to the GAMSAT. There are plenty of sources willing to sell MCAT questions, which is another good source of practice materials which can be purchased online. Similarly, the Graduate Management Admissions Test (GMAT) is a test used in the United States to select for applicants into graduate business programs, with some sections similar to the GAMSAT (while some are quite different) – this is another source of practice questions that you can purchase online. Just search Amazon and you will find many books of practice questions.

Preparation Courses for the GAMSAT

The GAMSAT body (ACER) does not recommend any specific preparation courses, and in fact says that 'some commercial preparation courses might provide misleading information or advice to candidates'. Preparation courses often charge large fees and pretend that they have 'secrets' on the GAMSAT that will help get you great marks. Although they are often extremely expensive (sometimes over $1,000), any practice is helpful, so consider one of these courses. With this in mind, many people do not do these courses and are still successful in gaining entry into medical school. These courses are often intensive (e.g., Monday to Friday from 5pm to 10pm) and claim that they teach you everything you need to know for the GAMSAT. No doubt, they are unable to teach you the course work from Year 11 and 12 physics, first year university chemistry and biology, essay writing and comprehension in five days! However, the preparation courses do well to cover the required material in the given time period. It is recommended that you cover all the material before attending the course – this way, it reinforces everything you have taught yourself, and you can ask questions about things you don't understand.

The Day before the GAMSAT

A few tips:

- Try to limit your study the day before the exam. You will perform better if you are rested and relaxed.
- Ensure that you have the right equipment for the GAMSAT.
- Set an alarm for the morning (and ask a family member or friend to set theirs too) giving yourself adequate time.
- Go to bed early, and avoid alcohol, coffee or anything which will keep you awake or interfere with your sleep

There is often nowhere to store personal items at the examination site, and as such I would recommend you bring as little as possible. Consider bringing a bottle of water as it is a long test and you don't want to get dehydrated.

Things you MUST bring to the GAMSAT:

- Your GAMSAT admission ticket.
- Photo identification (current drivers license or passport).
- Lead pencils (at least 3, because once the test has started you don't want to be sharpening broken or blunt pencils, or trying to borrow them from the examiners), preferably Medium–Soft Number 2 or HB.
- An eraser.
- Blue or black pens (at least 3, because it would be awful if your medical dreams were derailed by your only pen running out of ink during the essay section).
- A watch to monitor your timing.

Applicants who do not speak English as a first language may bring a printed bilingual dictionary for use in Sections 1 and 3. However, the pages should not be marked and there should be no sticky notes or other pieces of paper inside. If you wish to do this, make sure you show the dictionary to one of the examiners before the test starts.

On the Day of the GAMSAT

A few tips:

- Give yourself adequate time to get ready and to get to the examination site.

- Have a low glycaemic index breakfast (e.g., cereal, toast) to keep your energy levels up throughout the day.

- Double check that you have all the required equipment with you (i.e., admission ticket, identification, pencils etc.).

- Pack yourself lunch and snacks or bring money to buy food.

- Arrive early to the examination site and either take this time to relax before the examination or review your summaries.

- Answer every question from start to finish.

- If you have difficulty with a question, mark that question in your question book and come back to it at the end.

- Don't spend too long on any particular question – rather move on and answer more questions before you run out of time.

- Choose your answer by the process of elimination. Cross out those answers that you know are wrong and then you can begin to deduce which answer is most likely right. Even if you have to guess between the last two, you have improved your chances from 25 percent to 50 percent.

- Circle your answers on the question sheet as a draft, but don't forget to transcribe your answers onto your answer sheet straight away – do not leave this until the end!

- All of the questions in Section 1 ('Reasoning in Humanities and Social Sciences') and Section 3 ('Reasoning in Biological and Physical Sciences'), the GAMSAT are multiple choice, and they all have the same value. You improve your chances if you answer as many questions as possible, leaving none out - even if this means you have to guess a few towards the end if you are running out of time. Marks are not deducted for wrong answers, so answer every question.

- Section 2 ('Written Communication') requires quick, well-thought-out construction of an argument, with an equally well constructed counter-argument, all tied together neatly and finished within thirty minutes so you can move onto the next essay to do it all over again. Your essay writing books will teach you how to construct well argued essays, but it is also often helpful to spend 5 minutes to outline and plan your essay. This can be as simple as quickly writing your main arguments and counter-arguments on a spare piece of paper, as once you have those, you can write a suitable introductory paragraph, with an equally suitable conclusion. Unfortunately there is no secret to writing good essays apart from practice. If you practice and add in a time constraint of 30 minutes, you will soon be ready to handle the GAMSAT essays of Section 2.

- In Section 3 ('Reasoning in Biological and Physical Sciences'), many students do not have enough time to answer all of the questions. This is because there are a lot of difficult questions with limited time. So, you must work quickly through the paper, answering everything you can, and don't dwell on really hard questions – you can come back to these later! There is no point in spending five minutes working out a really hard question, as the extra time you have just taken means you have lost the time to answer two other easy questions. So, I recommend you quickly guess the really hard questions (or ones that will take you a long time to calculate the answer), go through the rest of the test answering all the easy questions you can, and if you have time, come back to the hard ones. Even if you do not finish this section, don't worry! Many students don't, and still get into medical school! It is supposed to be a hard test, so you shouldn't find it easy!

> '*I like that medicine is extremely diverse. There are countless fields that you can enter and there is something there for any inquiring mind. Furthermore, I anticipate a high level of job satisfaction. At the end of the day the profession is about improving people's lives.*'
>
> Dr Ed Campion, Intern, St Vincent's Hospital, Sydney

GAMSAT examiners take the exam very seriously, and you can be disqualified from the test (and possibly from sitting the GAMSAT in the future) if you are seen carrying:

- Stationery apart from a pencil and eraser
- Mobile phones
- Calculators
- Stopwatches
- Dictionaries
- Recording devices

- Food (unless you have a medical certificate indicating you need it for medical reasons)

- Bags

Further, you can suffer similar penalties if you lie during the registration process, copy any part of the test to take with you upon leaving, work on a part of the exam you have not yet been instructed to work on and give or receive assistance to or from others.

Now you have prepared for this test for months, so do not stress! You have put in the hard work, and it is about to pay off. Just keep calm, answer everything you can and you will surprise yourself.

Good luck!

'Be in an environment where you are inspired to learn and to understand disease processes, where change is actively supported. Be involved with a team that can have fun as they learn. Be around people who have high ethical values and inspire, get the job done well and are aware that life is very short. Make a difference. Being in the right environment with the right people at the same time is gold. Treasure those times.'

Professor Suzanne Anderson, Consultant Radiologist, Southern Health Radiology, Melbourne

'Make sure you are passionate about studying medicine, and if so, go for it! Try to make uni fun and don't worry about getting the top grades – a tutor of mine who is a consultant gastroenterologist at a major hospital failed his third year at uni and he has done pretty well for himself! If you don't get in straight out of school, study a related degree such as science or medical science – this will really help you further down the track.'

Emily Sutherland, High Distinction Student, Sixth Year Medicine, University of New South Wales

7 | Special Applicants

Mature Age Students

Mature age students who are not currently studying at university can apply to a graduate medical program (see Chapter 6: 'Graduate Entry into Medical School and the GAMSAT'). If you apply as a mature age student you must have completed an undergraduate degree of at least three years. If you do have a previous degree, most universities require that you graduated no more than ten years ago – if you graduated over ten years ago, contact your chosen medical school for more information. However, if you fulfil these criteria, see Chapter 8: 'The Application' for information on how to apply to medical school.

Graduate Entry into Undergraduate Programs

This mode of entry involves commencing a science degree at university, and either after the first year or after graduation, being allowed to enter the undergraduate medical degree at that university. However, few spots are offered (usually 2 to 10 places for this type of entry each year). This is offered at several universities, most notably:

- University of New South Wales: Students who have just finished their second year of a Bachelor of Medical Science (BMedSc) degree at the University of New South Wales may apply. After completion of your third year of your BMedSc, you will need to complete an honours year, and then are able to transfer into Year 4 of medicine. Admission into this program is based on the students average mark in their BMedSc, their UMAT score and an interview.

- University of Western Sydney: Students complete their first year of either Advanced Science, Advanced Medical Science or Advanced Natural Science at the University of Western Sydney, and then may apply for admission into the undergraduate medicine program. Admission into this program is based on their average marks in their first year, their UMAT and their performance in an interview.

- University of Tasmania: Students complete their first year of either a Bachelor of Biotechnology and Medical Research, Bachelor of Pharmacy, Bachelor of Science, Bachelor of Biomedical Science, Bachelor of Health Science or Bachelor of Environmental Science at the University of Tasmania, and then apply for admission into the undergraduate medical degree. Admission is based on their average marks during that year, having satisfied Year 12 prerequisites, and their UMAT score.

- University of Adelaide: Students in their first or second year at the University of Adelaide may apply. Applicants are selected via their university marks and an interview.

- Bond University: Applications for this program are lodged through the Queensland Tertiary Admissions Centre, and must include evidence of your results in high school chemistry, English and maths B. Contact the university for more information.

- Flinders University: Students complete 2 years of a Bachelor of Clinical Sciences, before entering the 4-year graduate medicine course. Applicants are selected via their high school and UMAT scores.

Indigenous Students

There are currently only 161 doctors who identify as Aboriginal and/or Torres Strait Islander in Australia. Several medical schools in Australia are attempting to rectify the imbalance in opportunity, offering alternate entry schemes to students who identify as Aboriginal and/or Torres Strait Islander.

Applicants can often apply directly to the medical school, so contact your chosen medical school. Great websites for indigenous students include the Australian Indigenous Doctors Association (www.aida.org.au/becoming. aspx) and Leaders in Indigenous Medical Education (LIME) Network (www. limenetwork.net.au).

The LIME Network Indigenous Pathways into Medicine online resource is designed to help future indigenous students determine which university will be the best fit for them as they study to become a doctor. The resource is an online, searchable database, designed to provide a first point of contact for indigenous school leavers, mature aged students and graduates who are looking to undertake medical studies. The resource provides a comprehensive, searchable database to compare all the medical courses in Australia and Aotearoa/New Zealand, including entry requirements, location and course duration. In addition, information about alternate entry pathways and preparatory courses for indigenous people is linked to each university where available. The resource also provides further information on assistance with scholarships, housing and finance whilst studying, and contact details for indigenous student support staff and LIME Reference Group members at each university. You can visit the LIME Network website to try out the resource for yourself, and determine the best path for you to become a doctor at www.limenetwork.net.au/pathways

Medical schools that offer alternate entry streams to Aboriginal and/or Torres Strait Islanders, and their entry requirements are as follows:

1. Undergraduate Medical Schools:

  a. <u>University of New South Wales</u>

    i. Applicants are selected via:

      1. Academic capability, which may include high school marks, TAFE or university marks, and other evidence of academic ability

      2. Communication and interpersonal skills, and a demonstrated desire to practice medicine (assessed at interview)

      3. Commitment to, and knowledge of indigenous health issues (assessed at interview)

    ii. Applicants must submit an application to the University Admissions Centre (UAC), at www.uac.edu.au

    iii. Applicants do not have to sit the UMAT.

    iv. Applicants who are successful at the interview must complete the 'Pre-medicine Program', which is a 4-week course commencing in December.

    v. Website: http://rcs.med.unsw.edu.au/rcsweb.nsf/page/Indigenous+Entry+into+Medicine

  b. <u>University of Newcastle/University of New England (Joint Medical Program)</u>

    i. Applicants are selected via:

      1. Academic capability, which may include high school marks, TAFE or university marks, and other evidence of academic ability

      2. Personal qualities (assessed at interview)

      ii.   Applicants do not have to sit the UMAT.

      iii.   Successful students will then sit the 1-week 'Pre-medicine Program', via the University of Newcastle.

      iv.   Website: www.newcastle.edu.au/joint-medical-program/indigenous-students/

  c. <u>University of Western Sydney</u>

      i.   Applicants are selected via:

          1.   Academic capability, which is assessed via high marks

          2.   Desire to study medicine and likelihood of succeeding in the course (assessed at interview)

      ii.   Applicants to not have to sit the UMAT, but it is helpful to do so.

      iii.   Applicants may apply via the UAC, or directly to the school of medicine.

      iv.   Website: www.uws.edu.au/medicine/som/applying_to_medicine/mbbs/indigenous

  d. <u>University of Adelaide</u>

      i.   Applicants are selected via:

          1.   Academic capability, which includes high school marks and the UMAT

          2.   The Medicine and Dentistry Oral Assessment (an interview)

          3.   Alternatively, applicants can apply directly via the Aboriginal Access Scheme and undergo the Aboriginal and Torres Strait Islander Programs Unit (the Wilto Yerlo) selection process, which involves testing and an interview

      ii.   Website: http://health.adelaide.edu.au/school_phcp/ypih/indigenous/

  e. <u>Monash University</u>

      i.   Does not have facilitated entry schemes for indigenous students, but indigenous applicants may apply to be considered for the Deans Indigenous List (DIL).

      ii.   Students on the DIL may be offered additional interviews, and may have certain study costs waived.

iii. Website: http://med.monash.edu.au/medical/central/entry-sche
mes.html#4

f. University of Queensland

  i. Applicants are selected via:

    1. Academic capability, which includes high school and UMAT marks

    2. Desire to study medicine (assessed at interview and via application form)

    3. Interview

  ii. Website: www.som.uq.edu.au/future-students/bachelor-of-medi
cine-bachelor-of-surgery-%28mbbs%29/mbbs-admissions/
aboriginal-and-torres-strait-islander-entry.aspx

g. Flinders University (Undergraduate Entry)

  i. Flinders University offers a unique undergraduate pathway. Students enrol in a Bachelor of Clinical Sciences, and after two years enter the 4-year MBBS program.

  ii. Applicants are selected via:

    1. UMAT

    2. High school marks

    3. Interview

    4. The Indigenous Application Scheme form, which includes questions on:

      a. Why you wish to enrol in the Bachelor of Clinical Sciences/ MBBS program at Flinders

      b. Your career expectations

      c. Your educational background

      d. Your relevant work experiences

      e. Your prior learning experiences

      f. Your community involvement

  iii. Website: www.flinders.edu.au/future-students/how-to-apply/spe
cial-entry/indigenous-access-scheme.cfm

h. Bond University

Does not have facilitated entry schemes for indigenous students.

i. James Cook University

Does not have facilitated entry schemes for indigenous students.

j. University of Tasmania

Students are recommended to identify as Aboriginal and/or Torres Straight Islander in their application form.

k. University of Otago

  i. Twenty places are set aside each year for Maori and Pacific Islander students.

  ii. Students must indicate their indigenous heritage on the application form.

  iii. Applicants are selected via:

    1. Academic marks (based on your performance in the Health Sciences First Year Program and the UMAT)

    2. Interview

  iv. Website: http://healthsci.otago.ac.nz/admissions/pp.html

2. Graduate Medical Schools

a. University of Sydney

  i. Applicants are selected via:

    1. Academic capability (GAMSAT and GPA – which may be less than those required for general entry, at the discretion of the dean)

    2. Interview

  ii. Website: http://sydney.edu.au/medicine/future-students/medical-program/domestic/indigenous-applicants.php

b. University of Notre Dame (Sydney)

There are no specific facilitated entry pathways for indigenous applicants, but applicants are encouraged to contact the School of Medicine directly (see Chapter12 for contact details).

c.   University of Wollongong

There are no specific facilitated entry pathways for indigenous applicants.

d.   University of Melbourne

There are no specific facilitated entry pathways for indigenous applicants, but applicants are encouraged to apply via Graduate Access Melbourne, at www.futurestudents.unimelb.edu.au/admissions/ applications/other-applications/how-to-apply. It is recommended that you contact the School of Medicine directly (see Chapter12 for contact details).

e.   Monash University

   i.   Applicants are selected via:

      1.   Academic capability, which includes university marks (i.e., GPA) and the GAMSAT

      2.   Interview

   ii.   Consider submitting a 'Centre for Australian Indigenous Studies' Supplementary Form.

   iii.   Applicants may be eligible to have certain study costs waived.

   iv.   Website: www.med.monash.edu.au/medical/central/entry-schemes. html#5

f.   Deakin University

There are no specific facilitated entry pathways for indigenous applicants, but applicants are encouraged to indicate they have an indigenous background on the GEMSAS application form.

g.   Flinders University

   i.   Applicants are selected via:

      1.   Academic capability (GPA)

      2.   Community involvement, desire to study medicine, and personal achievements (assessed via application form)

      3.   Interview

   ii.   Applicants are not required to sit the GAMSAT.

iii. Website: www.flinders.edu.au/medicine/sites/medical-course/domestic-applicants/indigenous-applicants.cfm_

h. Univeristy of Queensland

    i. Applicants are selected via:

        1. Academic capability, which includes high school and university marks

        2. Résumé, which includes referees and qualifications;

        3. Desire to study medicine (assessed at interview and via application form)

        4. Interview

    ii. Website: www.som.uq.edu.au/future-students/bachelor-of-medicine-bachelor-of-surgery-%28mbbs%29/mbbs-admissions/aboriginal-and-torres-strait-islander-entry.aspx

i. Griffith University

    i. Applicants are selected via:

        1. GAMSAT

        2. Academic marks (GPA)

        3. Interview

        4. Completion of the Alternative Entry Program Application form

    ii. Website: www.griffith.edu.au/gumurrii-student-support-unit/future-students/alternative-entry-program

j. University of Western Australia

    i. Alternative entry for indigenous students is considered on a case-by-case basis.

    ii. Applicants apply directly to the Centre for Aboriginal Medical and Dental Health.

    iii. Applicants are selected via:

        1. Academic marks (GPA)

        2. Résumé (including referees, qualifications and experience)

        3. Application form

        4. Interview

iv.   Applicants are not required to sit the GAMSAT.

v.   Website: www.meddent.uwa.edu.au/courses/postgraduate/apply-professional/indigenous-path

k.   <u>University of Notre Dame (Perth)</u>

There are no specific facilitated entry pathways for indigenous applicants, but applicants are encouraged to contact the School of Medicine directly (see Chapter12 for contact details).

l.   <u>Australian National University</u>

i.   Applicants are selected via:

1.   University marks – must be equivalent to 50 percent or greater

2.   Score within 10 percent of the mean GAMSAT mark for that year

3.   Interview

4.   Submitting a 'Supplementary Form: Indigenous Australian Admission Scheme' found at www.anu.edu.au/sas/forms/iaas.pdf

ii.   Website: http://medicalschool.anu.edu.au/programs-courses/bachelor-medicine-bachelor-surgery/how-apply/indigenous

Rural Students

Most medical schools have separate places for students with significant rural backgrounds. To determine whether a student has lived in a rural area, universities use the 'Australian Standard Geographic Classification (ASGC) Remoteness Areas' (see www.doctorconnect.gov.au/internet/otd/Publishing.nsf/Content/locator for rural locations). Universities consider a rural background to include rural areas (RA) 2 to 5, with the five categories being:

RA-1   Major city

RA-2   Inner regional

RA-3   Outer regional

RA-4   Remote

RA-5   Very remote

You must have lived in the rural area for 5 years (consecutively or cumulatively), since beginning primary school. To prove that you have lived in such an area for the requisite time, you must supply supporting documents which may include:

- School reports
- Transcripts from your university
- Supporting letters from a school, university or workplace
- Documents to prove residence (including bills for telephones/rates/utilities, or bank statements showing your address)

To find out if your chosen medical school offers such an avenue and you qualify, contact your chosen medical school.

International Students

Some universities accept international students, while others do not. Unfortunately, most places for international students are full-fee-paying, costing between $25,000 and $52,000 per year (see Chapter 8 for details). However, this means that many universities have set aside separate places for international students. International students may be subject to an English proficiency test. Some universities require that international students apply with either a UMAT or GAMSAT, while others require an ISAT score (International Student Admission Test for international students applying to Australian universities) or an MCAT score (Medical College Admissions Test, the admissions test for the United States and Canada), and some may require an International English Language Testing System (IELTS) score. The ISAT is a 3-hour multiple-choice exam administered by computer (http://isat.acer.edu.au/), while the MCAT is a 5-hour multiple-choice exam with sciences and comprehension (www.aamc.org/students/applying/mcat/).

Each medical school has a slightly different English-language requirement for overseas-born students: an IELTS score of seven is generally acceptable for medical school entry, but a score of seven or above is mandatory for Australian Health Practitioner Regulation Agency (AHPRA) registration. Unless you have completed high school certificate English, it will be necessary for you to complete an IELTS exam in the two years prior to completing medical school and being registered. (Further details may be found on the APRA website, www.ahpra.gov.au.)

The 'medical student tsunami' is likely to impact the provision of jobs for international students, so see Chapter 1, under the heading 'What it's Like to Become a Doctor'.

Universities that accept international students are listed below, along with entry requirements.

1. Undergraduate Medical Schools

a. University of New South Wales

    i.   Applicants will be selected via:

         1. High school mark equivalent to an academic rank of at least 96.00 (out of 100)

         2. Results of the ISAT

         3. Interview

    ii. Website: www.med.unsw.edu.au/medweb.nsf/page/Selection_Intl

b. University of Newcastle/University of New England (Joint Medical Program)

    The JMP does not offer places for international students.

c. University of Western Sydney

    i.   Applicants will be selected via:

         1. Academic capability (either a high school mark of 95.5 out of 100, or a GPA of 5.6 or higher out of 7 over a completed degree, or a GPA of 6.0 or higher over one year of a degree)

         2. ISAT results

         3. A good command of written and spoken English, assessed via either the IELTS (must score at least 6.5 in each section, or an overall score of 7.0), having completed 5 years of secondary education in English, or having completed the Higher School Certificate in Australia

         4. Interview

    ii. Website: www.uws.edu.au/medicine/som/applying_to_medicine/mbbs/international_applicants

d. Monash University

   i. Applicants are selected via:

      1. High school marks, equivalent to over 90 out of 100

      2. ISAT results

      3. A good command of written and spoken English, assessed via either the IELTS (must score at least 6.5 in each section, or an overall score of 7.0), or a Cambridge GCE O level.

      4. Interview

   ii. Website: www.med.monash.edu.au/medical/central/international.html

e. University of Adelaide

   i. Applicants are selected via:

      1. High school marks, equivalent to over 90 out of 100

      2. A good command of written and spoken English, assessed via an IELTS score of at least 6.5 overall

      3. Personal Qualities Assessment

      4. Structured Oral Assessment

   ii. Website: www.adelaide.edu.au/degree-finder/bmbbs_bmbbs.html

f. James Cook University

   i. Applicants will be selected via:

      1. Academic capability, which varies depending on country – requirements by country can be found at www.jcu.edu.au/international/entry/JCUPRD1_062728.html (Note that the UMAT is NOT required by James Cook; applicants must have at least an exit level 'Sound Achievement' in English, maths B and chemistry or equivalent)

      2. A good command of written and spoken English, assessed via an IELTS score of at least 7.0 overall, with 7.0 in three components

      3. Application form

      4. Interview

ii.   Website: www.jcu.edu.au/international/apply/JCUPRD_057105.
html

g.   Bond University

Bond University does not offer places for international students.

h.   University of Tasmania

   i.   Applicants will be selected via:

      1.   Academic capability, assessed via any of the following: MUFY: 95 percent (average best 4); Trinity FY: 95 percent (average best 4); UNSWFP: GPA 9.5; WAUFP: CPS 75; IB: 36 (including bonus points); GCE A Levels: AAA; STPM: AAA; UEC/MICSS: A1 average; Ontario Secondary School Diploma: 89; Indian CBSE/CICSE/All India State Board: 95 percent; Korean IKHCC: 3.7; Sri Lankan SLGCE: 15 (aggregate of best 3 at the higher level); South African Snr Cert: 32 (aggregate of 6 subjects at higher grade); or Thai Mattayom 6: 3.7

      2.   Having achieved an A grade in chemistry at Australian Year 12 level (or equivalent)

      3.   A good command of written and spoken English, assessed via either the IELTS (must score at least 7.0 in each section, with an overall score of 7.0), a sufficient Test of English as a Foreign Language (TOEFL) score, or 2 years of full time study with English as the spoken language

      4.   ISAT score with minimum overall percentile of 50 percent

   ii.   Website:www.international.utas.edu.au/static/HowtoApply/Appli cationsforMedicinePrograms-HowtoApply.php

2. Graduate Medical Schools

a.   University of Sydney

   i.   Applicants are selected via:

      1.   University marks, equivalent to a GPA of 5.5 out of 7 or greater

      2.   GAMSAT and/or MCAT results (applicants can choose whether they submit their GAMSAT or MCAT results)

      3.   Interview

b. Website: http://sydney.edu.au/medicine/future-students/medical-pro gram/international/international-admissions.php#requirements

c. University of Notre Dame (Sydney)

 The UND does not offer places for international students.

d. University of Wollongong

 i. Applicants are selected via:

 1. University marks, equivalent to a GPA of 5.0 out of 7 or greater

 2. GAMSAT and/or MCAT results (applicants can choose whether they submit their GAMSAT or MCAT results). Minimum GAMSAT results are 50 overall and 50 in each section, and minimum MCAT result is M and 24 overall (with minimum of M)

 3. Admission portfolio

 4. Interview

 ii. Website: www.uow.edu.au/gsm/futurestudents/international/ index.html

e. University of Melbourne

 i. Applicants are selected via:

 1. University marks – there is no minimum GPA

 2. GAMSAT or MCAT score – there is no minimum GAMSAT or MCAT score

 3. A good command of written and spoken English, assessed via either the IELTS (must score at least 6.0 in each section, or an overall score of 7.0), or a sufficient TOEFL score

 4. Interview

 ii. Website: http://medicine.unimelb.edu.au/study-here/md/application_ process/international

f. Deakin University

 i. Applicants are selected via:

 1. University marks, equivalent to a GPA of 5.0 out of 7

 2. GAMSAT or MCAT score – minimum GAMSAT score is 50 (with a minimum of 50 in each section), and minimum MCAT score is 8/8/M/8

3. A good command of written and spoken English, assessed via an IELTS score of at least 7.0 in the written and spoken section, and an overall score of 7.0

4. Completed International Supplementary Information Form

5. Curriculum vitae

6. Interview

ii. Website: www.deakin.edu.au/health/medicine/admission-intl-students.php

g. Flinders University

i. Applicants are selected via:

1. University marks, equivalent to a GPA of 3.3 out of 4

2. GAMSAT or MCAT score – minimum GAMSAT score is 60 (with a minimum of 50, 46 and 50 in sections 1, 2 and 3 respectively), and minimum MCAT score is 29

3. Interview

ii. Website: www.flinders.edu.au/medicine/sites/medical-course/international-applicants/

h. University of Queensland

i. Applicants are selected via:

1. University marks, equivalent to a GPA of 5.0 out of 7

2. GAMSAT or MCAT score – minimum GAMSAT score is 50 in each section), and minimum MCAT score is 8/8/M/8

3. A good command of written and spoken English, assessed via an IELTS score of 7.0 in each section, and an overall score of 7.0 – alternatively, you can sit one of the international English tests, and achieve the necessary score found on the 'Undergraduate Prospectus for International Students' page on the international student website below

ii. Website: www.som.uq.edu.au/future-students/bachelor-of-medicine-bachelor-of-surgery-%28mbbs%29/mbbs-admissions/international-student-applications.aspx

i. Griffith University

i. Applicants are selected via:

1. University marks, equivalent to a GPA of 5.0 out of 7

2. GAMSAT or MCAT score – minimum GAMSAT score is 50 in each section, and minimum MCAT score is 8/8/M/8

3. A good command of written and spoken English, assessed via an IELTS score of 7.0 in each section, and an overall score of 7.0

4. Interview

ii. Website: www.griffith.edu.au/health/school-medicine/future-students/admissions

j. University of Western Australia

i. Applicants are selected via:

1. University marks, equivalent to a GPA of 5.5 out of 7

2. GAMSAT or MCAT score – minimum GAMSAT score is 50 overall (and 50 in each section), and minimum MCAT score is 8/8/M/8

3. A good command of written and spoken English, assessed via an IELTS score of 6.0 in each section (and an overall score of 6.5), or one of the English proficiency exams listed at www.studyat.uwa.edu.au/undergraduate/admission/english

4. Interview

ii. Website: www.meddent.uwa.edu.au/courses/postgraduate/apply-professional/int-std-path

k. University of Notre Dame (Fremantle)

The UND does not offer places for international students.

l. Australian National University

i. Applicants are selected via:

1. University marks, equivalent to a GPA of 5.6 out of 7

2. GAMSAT or MCAT score – minimum GAMSAT score is 55 overall (and 50 in each section), and minimum MCAT score is 8/8/M/8

3. A good command of written and spoken English, assessed via an IELTS score of 7.0 in each section

4. Interview

ii. Website: http://medicalschool.anu.edu.au/programs-courses/bachelor-medicine-bachelor-surgery/how-apply/international

8 | The Application

1) *Decide medicine is for you*

2) *Position yourself:*

   a. *Optimise marks in high school or university*

   b. **Obtain extra-curricular experience**

3) *Study and sit for the entry exams (UMAT or GAMSAT)*

4) **Prepare and submit your application**

5) *Prepare for and sit your interview*

6) *Accept your invitation to medical school*

UMAT and GAMSAT scores are valid for two years, so you do not have to sit these tests each year before which you wish to apply. Keep in mind that university entry scores change each year, so you should choose your best score for your application – but if your marks were only enough to barely get an interview, you may want to re-sit the exam to improve your chances.

Each university has its own values, as well as its own individual benefits and drawbacks, so choose wisely. This chapter deals with which types of universities you should consider applying to (depending on your personal preferences), and how to tailor your application appropriately to maximise your chances. You have already put in the hard work with your school or university marks and the UMAT and GAMSAT, so make sure you put in the effort in your application!

Where to Apply?

Which university to apply to depends on where you live, your personal preferences, and how confident you are that you will get accepted.

Some people prefer to attend a medical school that is close to them, but others are happy to travel long distances, or even move across states to attend a medical school with a good reputation. It is your choice, but keep in mind – all medical schools are basically the same. Once you have graduated from medical school, no one cares which university you went to, so there may be no point in sacrificing your time or money just to go to a prestigious university.

Personal preferences have a large part to play in which university you apply to. For example, some universities such as Notre Dame have a religious foundation which some applicants may seek. Other universities such as Wollongong seek to train doctors to work in rural areas, while others have a research focus. As well as the values of the university, you must consider the individual benefits and drawbacks of the universities. Some universities have been around for years, are prestigious and place you at large teaching hospitals, but have large class sizes and the teaching may not be optimal. For example, they may have subjects taught by science researchers, rather than medical doctors. Some of the smaller universities may have great teaching and small class sizes, but lack the prestige and access to large teaching hospitals.

In doing your research on the various aspects of each university (some of which I have discussed at the back of this book), you will not only learn which university suits you best but you will also have some great material to talk about in the interview, to demonstrate why that specific university suits you well and to demonstrate how thoroughly you have researched that medical school. Another great idea is to attend course information sessions held by medical schools throughout the year – check your chosen universities website for more information.

How confident are you that you will be accepted? If your high school or university and entrance exam marks are fantastic and you interview well, you probably can choose whichever medical school you like best and they will accept you. However, if you have not achieved perfect marks or you aren't confident in your interview skills, you may need to consider what is more important to you – getting into a prestigious, highly sought after medical school or just getting into any medical school? The older, more prestigious universities have thousands of people apply to them, so they can afford to be more selective and getting into them is often more competitive. So unfortunately, you must also consider that if you are not 100 percent confident about your application being accepted, you may have to apply to your 'second choice' university – after all, isn't becoming a doctor more important than which university you went to?

It is important to remember that application forms are due at various times throughout the year (generally anywhere from May to September), so check your preferred medical school's website for specific dates.

The Application Form

Many medical schools require additional material before they will consider you for an interview. This often includes your curriculum vitae (CV) or résumé (see below) or a supplementary form which demonstrates your past achievements. Make sure that if this is required you tailor it to the specific university you are applying for. That is, research the values of each university and write your application appropriately – whether they are a university that focuses on research, rural medicine or anything else, ensure that you appeal directly to that university.

Try and distinguish yourself from the crowd. Every other applicant is smart, scored well at school and university and on the entrance exams (UMAT or GAMSAT). What makes you different? Why should they choose you over the others? If you can find out something special about the university it will show that you are interested and have done your research, as well as distinguish you from the other applicants. Include other details of your achievements or work that will set you apart from the other applicants.

If an application form is required rather than a CV, fill out the application form as if it is a CV, following the CV advice below (as most application forms require personal details, qualifications, achievements, extra-curricular activities and so on – just like a CV).

> 'Study hard and embrace your inner nerd, but don't forget there is life outside of medicine.'
>
> Dr Catherine Crane, Senior Resident, Concord Hospital, Sydney

Curriculum Vitae

Many medical schools require a curriculum vitae (or CV), which is an account of your past education, jobs and achievements. To present your best self, you must present a CV that details how your personality, characteristics and achievements are similar to those sought out in the medical profession. That is, that you are not just academically talented, empathic, a good leader and communicator, and a seasoned team player, but you also have other interests apart from study (i.e. other hobbies) and are therefore a balanced person. In order to prove you work well in a team, for example, it is good to show you have worked in many teams. Many books on writing a good CV are available from Amazon. Positions and situations you can put yourself in that will both look good on your CV and in your interview are found below. For sample CVs, see Appendix C. For more information on CV writing, see the ANZ Journal of Surgery website on CV writing at www.anzjsurg.com/view/0/writingACV.html, or the Seek website on CV writing at www.seek.com.au/jobs-resources/get-your-dream-job/resume-guide

How to Write a Curriculum Vitae

There are several ways to organise a CV, of which the chronological model is often the most effective for medical applications, as it is quick and easy to read (remember that the university staff will be reading hundreds of these). This involves structuring your CV as below, listing your achievements in reverse chronological order – that is, from most to least recent (for example, list your university degree before your higher school certificate). This allows the assessors to easily view your most recent (and therefore most relevant) academic achievements. Do not include everything you have ever done, as it can make your CV look cluttered and detract from the most important parts. For each achievement, consider whether it will contribute to your application before you include it.

While it may be tempting to make your CV as eye-catching as possible, keep it simple. Simple black text on a white background, with no pictures looks professional, and most importantly, is easy to read. As most CVs are sent electronically, make sure you have the correct file format (whether .doc, .docx, or .pdf). Microsoft Word has pre-made CV templates which are easy to use.

For most job applications, a CV is accompanied by a cover letter which outlines your desire and suitability for the position, but most medical schools do not require this. Similarly, some CVs include an 'overview' paragraph after your personal details, which summarises your achievements and outlines your ambitions and career goals – not all CVs have this, and it may not be necessary for an application to medical school (but will be necessary for later job applications!).

Your CV will obviously differ whether you are applying for undergraduate or graduate medicine (for example, if you are in high school you are unlikely to have an extensive work history, or a long list of publications).

Remember to update your CV regularly. In fact, whenever you achieve something worth placing on there, do it immediately. Things often slip your mind when writing your CV, and it is much easier to just keep it up to date.

For sample CVs, see Appendix C.

Conventional Curriculum Vitae Structure

<u>Personal Details</u>

Name

Address

Phone number (mobile number at minimum, consider including your home phone number) and email address.

While it was once expected to include your gender, age, ethnicity and/or religion, this is no longer necessary and may appear outdated. In fact, legislation exists to prohibit assessors taking such information into account.

<u>Qualifications</u>

List the qualifications you have achieved, along with the year and institution. Consider including your major, if a university degree. Include non-academic qualifications (such as first aid certificates, non-academic TAFE or Responsible Service of Alcohol qualifications). If you are part-way through study, write this as, for example, 'Higher School Certificate, 2012–current', or include the predicted completion date (e.g., 'Bachelor of Arts/Bachelor of Science 2011–2014').

<u>Work History</u>

Include the position you held, dates (e.g., February 2011–March 2012, or if still working, write it as, for example 'April 2011–current'), and a short summary of the position, including things you learnt. This summary should demonstrate skills and attributes relevant to your medicine application. For example, if you worked at a bar you would not write 'This role involved pouring beer and mopping the floor', but could instead state: 'This role involved working closely with others, and required excellent communication and teamwork skills. It was also physically demanding, and taught me the ability to multitask as well as prioritise.' Include more detail about your current or more recent job(s), with less detail for older ones.

<u>Publications</u>

If relevant, include any publications you have achieved (whether in a journal, book chapter, or newspaper or school/university newsletter).

List these in the format you would use to cite any publication (for examples, see the References section of this book).

Awards and Achievements

List your achievements. These can be as diverse as academic awards or scholarships, sporting awards, being captain of a sporting team, speaking another language, or being part of a winning debating team. Include anything which demonstrates the characteristics of a doctor mentioned in Chapter 2.

Extra-curricular Activities

This can include mentoring other students, volunteer work, or anything which demonstrates you have gone out of your way to help others and are committed to improving the quality of life of other people.

Referees

The selection panel may wish to contact people to verify your CV, or to find out more about you. This is achieved by you listing (often two) referees who are willing to be called and discuss you. Choose people who have seen you work (it is often better to include a boss than a co-worker), and who like you and are thus likely to say good things about you. You should check with your potential referees before listing them that it is OK you do so, and it is often helpful to tell them that you are applying for medicine.

Include: referee's name, their role, the company they work for and their contact details (phone number and email).

How to Best Present Your Characteristics

These are not only important to look good on your CV, sound good in the interview, or teach you necessary skills, but also to enforce good patterns of behaviour which you will need to maintain throughout your career. Medicine is highly stressful and demanding, so maintaining a balanced life is essential for survival.

Academic Qualities

Your academic prowess is already established by your ATAR (or equivalent) or GPA and UMAT or GAMSAT. However, it is also possible to stand out from others by demonstrating other academic achievements. These include:

- Being part of debating teams
- Studying a language
- Taking part in academic competitions – e.g. Maths/Physics/Chemistry/ Biology Olympiads, or International Competitions and Assessments for Schools Maths, Science, English, or Computer Skills Tests
- Achieving first place in subjects or classes at school or university
- While at university doing an honours year, or being part of a research group as a paid or volunteer researcher – this may give you the opportunity to get journal articles published, or appear at conferences

Leadership

The best way to prove you are a good leader is exactly that – to *prove* it. Therefore, it is essential you can give several examples of times you have had a lead role. Ideally, you would have leadership experience in several areas, not just at school, or just on the sports field, but a combination. Like all other characteristics, it is also helpful to demonstrate a history of this behaviour. Examples of leadership activities are being:

- Captain of a sporting team
- Student representative at school and/or university
- School/club captain
- Head of a debating team
- Coach of a younger team in sport or academic pursuits
- In a job which puts you in a lead role

Communication

For your CV and the interview, it is important you have notable communication experience (i.e. you have been involved in activities that require communication). Some ideas of such activities include:

- Being part of a debating team
- Attending Toastmasters, an organisation that helps people with public speaking (more detail on Toastmasters is found at their website, www. toastmasters.org.au) – this is also a great skill to have for the interview
- Being a student representative at school and/or university

- Having a part-time job that requires good communication (such as a personal trainer, waiter/waitress, hospital orderly or assistant-in-nursing)
- Being involved in a research group at university
- Being part of a sporting team where communication is important

Teamwork

Applicants often struggle with finding examples of their teamwork roles. It is also important in your application and interview to identify what kind of role you play in a teamwork situation and how your other characteristics come into play in a team (i.e. being an open communicator, active listener, mediating conflict, leading and so on). Examples of the kinds of teams you may have been part of include:

- Being part of a sports team
- Working in a cafe/restaurant/shop
- Being part of a debating team
- Working well in group assignments at school or university

Other Characteristics

Read the medical school's literature from their website and open days, and if possible, speak to students and staff. You will find that each university differs slightly in terms of what it seeks to achieve, and what it wants from prospective students. For example, the University of Notre Dame, Australia aims to produce leaders in medical care while the University of Wollongong aims to train practitioners willing to contribute in remote and rural communities. With this in mind, you may need to tailor your application to the specific school you are applying to. That is, if applying to a medical program with a focus on producing rural graduates, you need to demonstrate an interest in remote communities and rural health.

Medicine is physically and mentally demanding, so the selection panel is mindful to look for students that have interests outside of medicine. The selection panel want well-balanced people that have other interests besides medicine and are able to manage these with a stressful and demanding course and career. Other interests include playing a musical instrument, sport and paid work.

Volunteering suggests you are active in your community and willing to give to others, both characteristics sought in aspiring medical students. Completing the Duke of Edinburgh's Award (see www.dukeofed.com.au) is a good way to indicate that you posses all of these characteristics, as well as participating in volunteer work. Examples of volunteer work include:

- Volunteering at an aged-care facility or hospital (a great choice, as you are both in a medical environment and are interacting with people)
- Being a volunteer life guard at a beach or swimming pool
- Volunteering at a homeless shelter
- Volunteering with young children, at afterschool care for example
- Coaching a team sport
- Volunteering at camps for disabled children
- Volunteering to raise money for a donation to a community charity
- Volunteering with the Red Shield Appeal.
- Being a regular blood donor to the Red Cross

See the references for websites which help young people find volunteering roles.

Lying

Lying in your CV or application form (or even in the interview) is unacceptable. Sometimes you will get away with it, but why take that chance? For example, lying and saying you came first in a subject at high school or university seems harmless (especially if you just came second), but the academic world is very small, and they may know who taught that subject, and will find out it wasn't you that topped it! Or, if you say you volunteered at a homeless shelter while you did no such thing, they may get the urge to call up and check that out (they will often want a phone number so they can verify each claim) – and will discover that you are a liar. Even in the interview, would you want to risk a lie, on the rare chance that the interviewer's son or daughter actually came first in that subject and you will be found out? There is no need to embellish your application form or lie about achievements in your interview. Everyone has something different to offer. However, if you put a lie into your application you may be caught, and that lie will demonstrate to the assessors that you have no ethics and morals. One lie may undo the last 2 or 3 years of hard work – so don't risk it.

How to Apply

Applying to each medical school generally involves submission of an application form (which is often in the format of a summarised CV), evidence of your high school or university marks, and evidence of your admission test marks, accompanied by payment of an application fee.

Applications are submitted to each university in one of three ways:

- Direct to the university. This involves submitting your application form, along with evidence of your high school/university and entrance exam marks direct to the medical schools website.

- To the university *and* your local university admissions centre. The university admissions centres differ for each state, but include the University Admissions Centre (UAC) for NSW and the ACT, the Victorian Tertiary Admissions Centre (VTAC) for Victoria, the South Australian Tertiary Admissions Center (SATAC) for South Australia and the Queensland Tertiary Admissions Center (QTAC) for Queensland. These bodies organise undergraduate university admissions, determined by your high school certificate mark. Applications via the university and your local university admissions centre involve indicating your preference of medical school via the university admissions centre website, and submitting your application form to the university website.

- Directly to the Graduate Entry Medical School Admissions System (GEMSAS). The GEMSAS is the body which organises graduate medical school admissions for many universities; coordinating applications, interviews and offers. Applications involve indicating your preferences and uploading your application via the GEMSAS website. The GEMSAS website also has a helpful GPA calculator! You will post supporting documents to the GEMSAS.

- To the university *and* the GEMSAS. Applications involve indicating your preferences via the GEMSAS website and submitting your application form to the university website, with supporting documentation posted directly to the university.

As mentioned above, all applications occur online via the university, admissions centre or GEMSAS websites. The method of application to each medical school in Australia is listed below:

- Directly to the university:
  - Sydney University
  - University of Tasmania

- To the university *and* your local university admissions centre (indicated in brackets):
  - University of New South Wales (UAC)
  - University of Newcastle/University of New England (UAC)
  - University of Western Sydney (UAC)
  - Monash University (VTAC)
  - University of Adelaide (SATAC).
  - Bond University (QTAC)
  - James Cook University (QTAC)
- Directly to the GEMSAS:
  - University of Wollongong
  - Monash University (graduate entry)
  - Deakin University
  - Flinders University
  - University of Queensland
  - Griffith University
  - University of Western Australia
  - Australian National University
- To the university *and* GEMSAS:
  - University of Notre Dame (Sydney)
  - University of Notre Dame (Fremantle)
  - University of Melbourne

University Places and Fees

Different universities have a different number of places on offer for students and each place has a different fee structure. On application to each medical school, you list each place (e.g., Commonwealth Supported, bonded, full fee) in the order you would like to receive it, and the better you perform in your application (including high school or university and entrance exam marks) and interview, the more likely you are to receive your chosen place. The places and fees are not means tested. Contact your chosen medical school (see Chapter 12: 'University Information' for contact details of each university), and see http://studyassist.gov.au/sites/StudyAssist/ for more information.

The fee structures include:

- Commonwealth Supported Places – These places used to be known as HECS places, and are places in which the government subsidises the cost of studying. As medicine is Band Level 3, the direct cost to the student is around $9,408 per year.

- Bonded Places – These places make up 25 percent of all medical school spots for students, and students accepting one of these places must commit to working in an area of workforce shortage. This means that if an area is short of medical staff trained in a certain area, the students will be sent there once they are qualified, as part of their agreement. The government will subsidise your fees, so the cost will be the same as for a Commonwealth Supported Place (around $9, 408) – the only drawback is the commitment to work in an area of need. The number of years spent in these areas is equal to the length of their medical degree (for example, a 6 year degree means you will spend 6 years in these areas). For at least some of these years, the applicant will need to have finished their training – so you cannot just spend your whole 4 or 6 years in a workforce shortage or rural area while you are an intern or resident, you will instead have to spend some of your time in these areas once fully trained as a specialist. See http://www.health.gov.au/bmpscheme for more information.

- Medical Rural Bonded Places – The Rural Bonded Places are similar to the Bonded Places, but the applicant will be sent to rural or remote areas, not just metropolitan areas of need. However, the applicant is given $25,013 annually by the government, in 10 equal monthly instalments from March to December. Students are required to pay their HECS-HELP debt ($9,408 per year).

- Full-fee-paying places – You will pay the full cost of studying medicine, with no government subsidy. This is between $25,000 and $52,000 per year, depending on the university (see Chapter 12 for costs at each university).

On your application to a specific medical school, you must list in order of priority which of these places you will accept. Generally, a Commonwealth Supported Place is the most preferable, with a full-fee-paying place being the least preferred.

However, you must ask yourself – if I am offered a Bonded or Rural Bonded or full-fee-paying place, will I accept it? Will I be able to afford a full-fee-paying place, or will I actually want to go to the country to fulfil my obligations for a

Rural Bonded Place? These are questions worth thinking about, and discussing with friends and relatives.

You can defer your payments through the Australian taxation system (the money owed is then called the HECS-HELP debt), which will slowly begin taking out a small percentage of your income to repay your fees once you start earning a certain level of income per year (for 2012–2013, that amount is $49,096). This is done by filling out the form provided with your yearly fees invoice. The debt does not accumulate interest. The amount of interest that is paid on your HECS-HELP debt is seen below:

Repayment Income	Repayment Rate
Below $49,096	Nil
$49,096 – $54,688	4.00%
$54,689 – $60,279	4.50%
$60,280 – $63,448	5.00%
$63,449 – $68,202	5.50%
$68,203 – $73,864	6.00%
$73,865 – $77,751	6.50%
$77,752 – $85,564	7.00%
$85,565 – $91,177	7.50%
$91,178 and above	8.00%

Table taken from http://studyassist.gov.au/sites/studyassist/payingbackmyloan/loan-repayment/pages/loan-repayment

Remember that if you pay all of your fees up front (that is, at the beginning of each academic year), you will receive a 10 percent discount off your fees that year. Alternatively, if you make voluntary repayments (which you may do at any time), you will receive a bonus of 5 percent in addition to the value of your payment.

9 | The Interview

1) Decide medicine is for you

2) Position yourself:

    a. Optimise marks in high school or university

    b. Obtain extra-curricular experience

3) Study and sit for the entry exams (UMAT or GAMSAT)

4) Prepare and submit your application

5) **Prepare for and sit your interview**

6) Accept your invitation to medical school

Dress Code

The dress code for the interview is often a stressful concept for many students. Everyone knows that you should dress smartly, but what if you wear the wrong colour tie, or the wrong style of shoes? I had an 'interview consultant' tell me that the tie I wore to the interview the previous year was wrong, and I needed to go out and buy one completely different. If only I'd known it doesn't matter. Yes, it is important that you are well groomed, but small issues like cuff-link design, tie pattern, skirt colour and earring choice make no difference to the interview panel.

It is essential that you are well groomed and well presented, however as long as you are dressed conservatively and appropriately the interview panel will not be interested in the colour scheme of your outfit.

For women, this means a smart dress or a suit, or a conservative skirt and top with sensible shoes (not 6 inch heels). For men, this means a business shirt, suit pants and leather shoes. For graduate entry medicine, a suit jacket and tie are mandatory, but they may not be appropriate for an undergraduate interview. However, it is better to be overdressed than underdressed, so I would recommend you wear a tie and suit jacket to any medical school interview – you can always put the tie in your pocket and hang your suit jacket over the chair if you feel overdressed. Jeans are never OK.

Additionally your hair should be appropriately cut, no facial piercings (earrings are OK for women), clean shaven (guys) and smartly dressed. A good rule of thumb is to dress like an accountant or lawyer, and a good test is to look in the mirror and ask 'Do I look like a doctor?'

> *'Be honest at the interview. Always dress as if you are attending patients on the wards. A tie is safer than an open neck shirt. It is easy to make a bad impression when you think that you are making a statement about being casual. For girls – no bum crack or cleavage! No matter how good you think it might be.'*
>
> Associate Professor Ray Garrick, Consultant Neurologist, St Vincent's Hospital, Sydney

I have heard a lot of people say 'I'm going to wear my hair uncut/dreadlocks/piercings' or 'I'm going to show off my tattoos', since 'I don't care who they think they are, I'm just going to be myself'. The interview panel are trying to gauge whether you look like a doctor – this means dressing slightly conservatively and not giving them a reason not to like you. Small matters like choice of tie (unless it is a novelty tie) or colour of skirt do not make a difference, since they are there to decide if you act like a doctor. With this in mind, if you are too 'out there' for their taste (for example, long-uncut hair or piercings on males, cleavage or short skirts on females) you may be sabotaging your chances. These may be very superficial, outdated views, but do you really want to risk it?

Many people have not spent much time in business clothes, so often look and feel uncomfortable in them. It is worth getting used to your interview clothes, so you look comfortable and relaxed to the interview panel. The last thing you want to be doing in your interview is thinking about how strange you feel in your clothes, rather than thinking about the ethical dilemma they have just posed you. Be sure to get other people's opinions on your interview clothes.

> *'I was pretty nervous. It is the last step before gaining entry into medicine so it's a very important day. Luckily the interview itself was surprisingly relaxed.'*
>
> Dr Ed Campion, Intern, St Vincent's Hospital, Sydney

How to Prepare for the Interview

You will be facing a panel of 1 to 5 interviewers, and the interview will go from 8 to 60 minutes.

My first suggestion to you is ask yourself – is there anything that would prevent you being completely confident in talking to an interview panel? This may include shyness, lack of self confidence and fear of public speaking. If so, address that immediately – this may involve joining Toastmasters (see their website in the References section), or getting a job or volunteering position which forces you to interact with people on a regular basis.

Next, practice the type of questions they will be asking. There are several pages of examples in Appendix D, but they are all variations on a theme. They are either about you (for example, 'Why do you want to be a doctor?', 'Why would you be a good doctor?'), or about how you would handle certain situations (for example, students cheating on an assignment, stressful jobs, angry patients).

In addition, the interviewers may want to know what your good qualities are, but also what your character flaws are, which parts of your personality you wish you could change – and what are you doing about it?

It is helpful to keep a notebook where you jot down ideas, examples and questions you have about these issues. For example, make a long list of things that would make you a good doctor (and a hopefully much shorter list of things that might make you struggle to be a good doctor – and how you can fix them).

> *'They know you are nervous, just try to be yourself and be as natural as possible. Don't make things up and don't use scripted answers – half the reason they do interviews is simply to assess how you communicate with other people so smile and relax!'*
>
> Anika Johnston, High Distinction Student, Sixth Year Medicine, University of New South Wales

Do not get too worried about trying to sound original. It is definitely helpful to differentiate yourself from others, but by saying something stupid just to get noticed you may be ruining your chances of admission. For example, don't just say 'I want to cure cancer' unless you can back it up with a well reasoned explanation. Also try to demonstrate ways in which you possess those all-important characteristics.

I can't tell you exactly what answers they are looking for, because I don't know. In fact, there is no perfect answer that will guarantee you a spot in their medical school. What they are looking for is you to give examples of those important 'doctor like' characteristics; academic qualities, empathy, communication, teamwork and leadership. You may not be asked a question directly on this, so try to ensure you mention your characteristics when possible.

The interview will also address more general and worldly issues such as 'What are the problems with putting more money into anti-smoking education?' To effectively answer these types of questions it is important that you address both sides of argument, having appropriate information to call on, and weighing up pros and cons of an issue.

> *'Attempt to anticipate questions to the extent that you know roughly how to respond. You don't want to rehearse and sound like a robot, but you need to think very hard about why you have chosen a career in medicine and be able to answer the question sincerely and coherently.'*
>
> Dr Ed Campion, Intern, St Vincent's Hospital Sydney

To prepare for this section it will be useful to purchase medical ethics textbooks (marked with an asterisk in the References section) which will introduce you to some of the classic dilemmas of medical ethics and will give you a framework for dealing with these situations (as well as the most ethical way of dealing with them, and how and why this differs from the real world – things they love to hear in the interview). Reading the newspaper is another great way to get various opinions on medical and ethical quandaries, as well as current examples to drop during your interview – and it is likely they will ask you about current health or people-related issues. See the chapters in Gordian Fulde's book *Emergency Medicine: The Principles of Practice* on 'Rural and Indigenous Emergencies' and 'Emergency Department Administration, Legal matters and Quality Care' for an outline of rural and indigenous health, and legal issues in medicine.

Be familiar with the values in medical ethics. There are 6, although the first 4 listed below are the traditional values in medical ethics (see the references for medical ethics textbooks), and you should try and consider each of these in your interview:

- Beneficence – act in the best interest of the patient
- Non-maleficence – the well-known 'do no harm'
- Autonomy – respect the decision making capacity of the patient
- Justice – maintain fairness in distribution of resources

- <u>Dignity</u> – treat the patient and those around him/her with respect
- <u>Honesty</u> – be truthful, and always make sure that all consent begins with the patient being informed about a treatment

Once you have an idea about these issues, practice in your head about how you would answer the questions they would ask. For example, if asked the question 'Outline the pros and cons for euthanasia', try and include at least three of these in each answer.

Many questions also involve either cultural differences or social differences. It would be helpful to read up on the main cultural differences that cause issues in medical practice, as well as the social injustices that affect medicine. For example, traditional Hindu women feel incredibly uncomfortable having a male gynaecologist (Iyengar 2008). However, many cultures feel offended that people stereotype, for example, assuming that all Muslims would be incredibly upset and offended if accidentally fed pork – some maybe, but not all. Thus, it is best to talk to the patient (or 'patient' in your scenario) and establish the extent of their religious beliefs, before continuing to ascertain what you can do to assist them. On that note, talking to your patient is the most important thing you can do in these situations, and should be your first port of call. For example, if there is a Jehovah's witness who is refusing a blood transfusion (as they have the right to do if they are above 16 years old in New South Wales), discuss with them whether they would consider other types of transfusion (e.g., albumin, fresh frozen plasma and so on), as recent changes in the Watchtower (the Jehovah's Witness publication) allow certain types of transfusion – and it is by talking to them that you can resolve this. Social injustices play a big part in medical practice, and it is likely you will be questioned on ways to improve social justice or asked to list current social injustices.

Once you are confident with your answers, start writing them down in question and answer format, and practice having people ask you the questions. Also, get them to ask you any questions they can think of that you may be asked in the interview. This will often force you to think about issues you had never considered, which they will almost certainly do in the interview. I highly recommend practicing with friends and family, getting them to ask you questions so you become proficient at thinking on the spot, forming your answers and getting rid of any nervousness. Another good technique is to find some family friends who you do not know especially well, and get them to ask you some interview-style questions. This works especially well as you will not feel comfortable and will feel unfamiliar with them, just as you will feel with the interviewers on the interview panel.

The whole process of preparing for an interview is to increase your level of confidence and ensure you that you will be able to handle any question they may throw at you. There is a good chance they will ask you some of the questions you have practiced (so make sure your 'Why I want to be a doctor' answer is perfect), but there is an infinite number of questions they can ask you. The idea is that no matter what they have asked you aren't shocked or surprised, because you have some framework of answering the question and can give a smattering of examples from your five main doctor-like characteristics (see Chapter 2: 'Characteristics of a Doctor' and 'How to Best Present Your Characteristics' in Chapter 8: 'The Application').

In the Interview

In the interview you need to act professionally – be well spoken and do not use slang. Doctors are well educated and well spoken, and they will be expecting you to present this way. Consider each question, and once you have a well-thought-out answer, speak slowly and clearly. It is worthwhile to take a few seconds before responding to think about your answer – and definitely better than jumping in with a half-thought-out answer.

Try to use examples of your doctor-like characteristics (see Chapter 2 and Chapter 8) as well as consider the six values in medical ethics, and do not forget to offer both sides of an argument – that is, if asked about euthanasia, don't just talk about the benefits, but also say 'on the other hand, I understand that there are some drawbacks…'

'I remember being pretty nervous, but I had lovely interviewers who made me feel at ease. They asked me all the questions you would expect: "Why do you want to be a doctor, what makes a good doctor, why would you make a good doctor etc." – I think it is a good idea to have a think about these ideas but don't rehearse answers because I'm sure they can tell!

I tried to make my answers as personal as I could – try to think about the real, deep reasons behind why you do want to be a doctor and don't just use the old "I want to help people!" I think it helps if you can make it specific to yourself and your own life.

My interviewers also asked me some more left-field questions that I wasn't expecting – it is perfectly OK to say "That's a hard question… Do you mind if I have a minute to think about that?"'

Anika Johnston, High Distinction Student, Sixth Year Medicine, University of New South Wales

'*Be yourself! Relax, they aren't there to give you bad marks – these people are trying to fill places in the degree. Be honest with your answers and try to seem enthusiastic about the idea of studying medicine and being a doctor.*'

Emily Sutherland, High Distinction Student, Sixth Year Medicine, University of New South Wales

There are 2 main types of interview, with different universities employing different interview types:

- Interview Panel: You will be interviewed by two or three interviewers who will ask you questions, and you will be able to respond in your own time. While this interview style carries less stress than the MMI (see below), if you make a mistake you have to pick yourself up and go on – you are stuck with these interviewers for the whole interview! Universities that use this style of interview are:

    o University of New South Wales

    o University of Adelaide

    o University of Notre Dame (Sydney)

    o University of Western Australia

    o Flinders University

    o University of Notre Dame (Fremantle)

    o Australian National University

    o University of Otago

- Multi-station Mini Interview (MMI): This style involves the candidate being asked questions by separate interviewers in separate interview stations. That is, you generally wait outside a closed door and once a buzzer sounds, you enter the door and are asked questions by a single interviewer until another buzzer sounds, at which point you then leave the room to wait for your next station. There are usually around 8 stations, each taking 8 minutes. This can be stressful, but the good news is that if you make a horrible mistake in one station; you have 7 other stations in which to make a good impression and make up for it! Universities that use this style of interview are:

    o University of Sydney

    o University of Newcastle/University of New England (Joint Medical Program)

- University of Western Sydney
- Monash University
- Bond University
- James Cook University
- University of Wollongong
- University of Melbourne
- Monash University
- Deakin University
- Griffith University

Neither Queensland University nor the University of Tasmania interview medical school applicants.

Practice interview questions are found in Appendix D.

'Political correctness is fairly easy to identify and expressions of fundamentalist, left-wing or right-wing philosophy are best left for the pub or the pulpit but not for the interview.'

Associate Professor Ray Garrick, Consultant Neurologist, St Vincent's Hospital

'I did two interviews – one whilst in Year 12 and one during uni. The first one was scary, especially as all the other kids waiting for their interviews went to selective schools. The second one was cruisy, although there was one nice and chatty interviewer and one who was expressionless (good cop, bad cop).'

Emily Sutherland, High Distinction Student, Sixth Year Medicine, University of New South Wales

10 | The Letter

1) *Decide medicine is for you*

2) *Position yourself:*

    a.   Optimise marks in high school or university

    b.   Obtain extra-curricular experience

3) *Study and sit for the entry exams (UMAT or GAMSAT)*

4) *Prepare and submit your application*

5) *Prepare for and sit your interview*

6) ***Accept your invitation to medical school***

Acceptance

Congratulations! You have worked hard for it, so enjoy your moment! Now is a great time to thank your family and friends for supporting, encouraging and putting up with you throughout the whole ordeal.

The only thing left to do now is accept the offer. Do this as quickly as possible (after reading all the information they send you), before they think you are not interested and give your spot to someone else!

See Chapter 11: 'You've Made it to Medical School!' for information on what medical school is like, and how to maximise your experiences and marks.

Rejection

What Now?

'It is with great regret that we inform you that you have been unsuccessful in your application to Medical School X for next year's intake.'

Receiving a letter or email like this is disappointing and upsetting. If you are like most medical school applicants then you are a habitual high achiever, who has rarely failed at anything in your life. Further, this is something you really want and have wanted for a long time, and it seems like all the hard work and dedication has been for nothing.

First of all, let me assure you that being unsuccessful in your medical school application doesn't mean you would make a bad doctor or are a bad person. As medical school selection criteria is currently very controversial, studies have examined how accurately the selection process correlated with academic performance and clinical skills (Groves 2007, Wilkinson 2008). They found that both GAMSAT and interview scores had no correlation to how good a medical student you were, from both an academic and clinical perspective. In fact, even the student's average mark from their first degree showed only a loose relevance.

What this means is lack of success in your application, whether you didn't make the cut due to your high school or university marks, UMAT or GAMSAT score, or performance in the interview doesn't mean you would be a bad medical student, or a bad doctor. In fact, because of the unreliability of the selection process, some US medical schools select students via completely random means. There are doctors who got into medical school on their first attempt, but many had to apply a second (myself included), or even third time.

It is understandable to be faced with an array of questions such as 'Should I apply again?', 'Will I be rejected a second time?', 'What will I do next year whilst I go through the application process again?', 'What will I do if I get rejected a second time?' and 'What other career options do I have?' It is important to reassess if you really want to get into medical school, and if this is something that you truly want to do, then you need it give it your all and try again.

I would go as far to say that after being rejected the first time, getting in the second time was so much sweeter! Overall, if I had to do everything again, I would do it exactly the same – right down to missing out on medical school the first time. It gave me a chance to reassess my life, decide I really did want to do medicine, have some time off and learn some things along the way.

> 'Never ever give up.'
>
> Associate Professor Nigel Hope, Consultant Orthopaedic Surgeon, Sydney Adventist Hospital

Rather than dwelling on your failure (which you will do enough of anyway, trust me) it is better to be proactive and focus on how you can improve your chances for next time. How to achieve this is covered later in the chapter.

Trying Again

You have considered it, and decided medicine is the only path for you. You have also realised that something wasn't right last time, and so you are going to address that problem and get in. For example, you may be amazing academically but your interview skills are not equally adept. On the other extreme, you may be a people person and scored top marks in your interview, but your school or university marks just weren't good enough to make the cut. It could also be a lack of experience working in a team, or perhaps you hadn't done enough volunteer work to wow the selection panel. Whatever the reason, it is important that it is identified and dealt with. This will require some quite honest introspection on your behalf, as well as from family and friends. You will need to identify those weaker areas in your application, interview and grades and if possible try to rectify or improve on them.

Your strategy for entering medical school after an initial failure differs whether you are an undergraduate or graduate student.

Undergraduate

You have applied for medical school during your last year of high school and have not been successful. It may not seem like it, but this is OK! As a recent school leaver you have plenty of time to reassess your path, and start preparing your new plan of attack. Your three options are:

1. Reapply for undergraduate medicine through UAC/QTAC/SATAC/VTAC/TISC;
2. Complete a degree at university before applying for graduate medicine;
3. Complete a degree at university before applying for graduate entry into undergraduate medicine.

Reapplying for undergraduate medicine next year is a valid option. I have several friends who missed out on medical school the first time around, but reapplied the following year and got into the medical school of their choice. One of my good friends actually got into medical school first go but didn't enjoy that particular school, so quit his studies at that university and reapplied through UAC for next year's entry – and was accepted to the medical school of his choice. Reapplying for undergraduate medicine will require you to wait until next year's application process, so you will need to decide what to do with yourself for a year. One option is to take a year off, recover from high school, earn some money and focus on your UMAT and application. Another option – possibly a safer option in the long term – is to begin a degree at university. This way if you don't get in to undergraduate medical school when you reapply the following year, you are already part way through a university degree which will open many doors for you, as well as give you the option to sit the GAMSAT and apply for graduate medicine.

Applying for graduate entry into an undergraduate medical program may mean that you will need to finish your current degree before doing so, or even just complete 1 year of that degree before transferring across into medicine (see 'Graduate Entry into Undergraduate Programs' in Chapter 7: 'Special Applicants' for more information).

These are some very important decisions to be made at this point in life, so it is crucial you get advice from others – including family, friends and career advisors.

> *'Develop resilience. This is something I sometimes see is lacking amongst students. Medicine requires a commitment to the profession which may mean a move, a change in circumstances or difficult placement. Be flexible and adaptable.'*
>
> Dr Elspeth Fotheringham, General Practitioner, Tuggerah

Graduate medical courses require you to have at least a bachelors degree in any area. Ideally you would have listed medicine-related degrees as fallback options when filling in your preferences – these include a Bachelor of Science, Bachelor of Medical Science, Bachelor of Pharmacy, Bachelor of Physiotherapy, Bachelor of Optometry or a Bachelor of Nursing, just to name a few (see below). These will give you a chance to learn related subjects, so will not only provide you with a strong base for your medical school education, but will prepare you for sitting the GAMSAT later on. However, it is also important you enjoy your undergraduate degree, and almost half of graduate medical students undertake non-science degrees such as architecture, engineering, arts and law. In fact if you enjoy your studies, you are more likely to do well and achieve a high Grade Point Average, which is an important criteria for graduate selection. I know several people who missed out on entry to medical school straight out of high school and did a combined science–arts degree in order to be best prepared for sitting the GAMSAT (since the GAMSAT is part science and part essay writing and comprehension).

There are other things to consider when choosing your backup degree. If you are unsuccessful in obtaining a place in graduate medical school, will you be happy to continue to study and work in the area of your undergraduate degree? For example, there is no point in choosing a history degree because you consider it to be easy to score highly, then missing out on medical school and having a qualification in an area you do not wish to continue in. The length of the degree is also important. If your goal is to get into medicine as soon as possible, undertaking a 3-year Bachelor of Science degree will (in the best case scenario) get you into medicine sooner than a 5-year combined Bachelor of Laws–Bachelor of Commerce. Although this may seem like a 'shallow' criterion, keep in mind that medical school is 4 years minimum, so you will be studying at university for 7 years if you choose the shortest degree – not to mention the years of study you will take on after graduating.

At this point, it may benefit you to read Chapter 6: 'Graduate Entry into Medical School and the GAMSAT'. This chapter deals with how to enter medical school after completing your university degree.

Graduate

After completing your first degree, you have applied for medical school and been unsuccessful. You may feel like you have failed again, or that you are running out of time – I mean, you are in your early twenties, and those who got straight into medical school from high school are almost finished! This is certainly not the case. You already have a degree under your belt and are old enough to have made the mature decision that medicine is the life for you. You now have two options for getting into medical school:

1. Reapply for graduate medicine

2. Sit the UMAT and apply for undergraduate medicine or graduate entry into undergraduate medical courses

> '*Only do this if you really know that you want to! There are many wonderful, enriching things about a life in medicine but there are some significant downsides. Medicine requires significant sacrifices and inevitably at times the balance of life will shift heavily towards work and study. There is a lot to learn and doctors work long, difficult hours. Study is endless and even after graduating it will continue. This concept of life-long learning is very appealing but imagine finishing a gruelling week only to spend the entirety of your days off studying for your next set of looming exams… Just some food for thought.*'
>
> Dr Ed Campion, Intern, St Vincent's Hospital Sydney

Your GAMSAT results are valid for 2 years, which means you can reapply without re-sitting the GAMSAT. However, if you missed out on an interview the first time around, this may be because your GAMSAT marks were too low to enable you to make the cut. If you did get an interview but were knocked back, this may be because your GAMSAT marks were not high enough. It is up to you whether you re-sit the GAMSAT, but it is definitely something I would recommend. You are at an advantage sitting the GAMSAT for a second time because you know the format of the exam, what the questions are like, what the timing is like, which study techniques suited you and which were your weaker areas. As such, it is likely that re-sitting the GAMSAT will enable you to increase your score. This is why I recommend sitting the GAMSAT in both the second-last and last year of your degree, so you have one year of practise, getting to know what to expect, and then a chance to do better.

If you do choose to re-sit the test, first sit down and write down what you could have done better last time, and resolve to do these things this time. I had done fairly well in comprehension and the sciences during my first GAMSAT, but could have done better in essay writing and organic chemistry. So, the second time around, I focussed on these two topics and could concentrate my efforts better as I knew what type of questions to expect. If you decide you could not have done any better on the GAMSAT and are not going to waste your time, that is fine – but don't rest on your laurels. Instead, start preparing your application, CV and honing your interview skills.

Several universities offer graduate entry into their undergraduate courses (see Chapter 7: 'Special Applicants'). This can take some planning, as graduate entry into undergraduate medicine is different to entry into graduate medicine. Criteria for graduate entry to undergraduate courses can be based purely on university marks, high school marks or a combination of the two. You must also sit the UMAT (Chapter 5: 'Undergraduate Entry into Medical School and the UMAT' for more information) and score well to be considered. You will need to prepare and study for the UMAT since the content is very different to what you have been doing in your university degree. You must also apply through your state's undergraduate university organisation, often as well as to the medical school to which you wish to go.

Applying for undergraduate study is not only a great backup plan for those applying to graduate medicine, but something which can teach you the skills needed to be successful in your graduate application.

At this point in your life, you can also consider taking a year off. After finishing my honours year, I had planned to go straight into graduate medicine. When this did not happen, I decided that taking a year off to focus on studying for and sitting the UMAT and GAMSAT would be beneficial, and this would also give me a chance to earn some money, as well as learn key skills I was missing, which may have caused me to miss a place in medical school. There is no rush in getting into and getting through medical school, as graduate medical students are on average in their mid to late twenties, and I know a successful doctor who now teaches at Harvard Medical School who entered medical school while in his forties. A year off may also give you time to do better in the medical entry tests, as well as giving you time to better yourself as a prospective doctor and just have some down time – especially after the pressure and stress of the previous few years.

Alternate Careers

There are many other careers that are likely to be just as rewarding. Many involve the medical sciences and working with others, and require a high degree of aptitude. They are all closely related to medicine, and you will often be working in a medical environment. At worst, they give you a fun, interesting few years before you decide to reapply to medicine!

Consider these careers:

- Nursing
- Physiotherapy
- Dentistry
- Dietetics
- Optometry
- Pharmacy
- Speech pathology
- Social work
- Occupational therapy
- Veterinary science
- Research/teaching

11 | You've Made It into Medical School

Congratulations! Now the real hard work begins!

> 'Work hard but not at the expense of doing other things that you enjoy – sport, seeing friends, reading, music, whatever. I know it's a cliché but balance is important and there is no point in achieving amazing marks if you have sacrificed everything else and become a less well-rounded person.'
>
> Anika Johnston, High Distinction Student, Sixth Year Medicine, University of New South Wales

This chapter outlines what your years at medical school are going to be like, and suggests some tips to help you study, as well as how to get the most out of your medical degree – because you must remember (although you have been ignoring this for the past few years in order to get in) that there is more to life than medicine!

Most medical schools divide their medical degrees into pre-clinical and clinical years.

Pre-clinical years: The pre-clinical years are usually the years in the first half of your degree, in which you spend most of your time in lectures and tutorials, poring through textbooks and learning the basics of the medical sciences.

Clinical years: The clinical years are those in which you spend some, and usually most of your time in hospitals (often called 'on placement') rotating through various specialties (for example, cardiology, general surgery, neurology, obstetrics and psychiatry just to list a few), and most of your actual study is with a textbook in your own time, plus a few hours of lectures and tutorials.

This chapter is divided to deal with each of these separately, as the study techniques for your pre-clinical and clinical years differ slightly. Be prepared – the years of medical school have been best years of my life so far!

Learning medicine is a step by step process, in which you add new pieces of information to ones you already have, building until you get the entire picture.

As I mentioned earlier in the book, you cannot know which medicine you should use to treat a disease (the pharmacology) unless you understand the anatomy (where things are in the body), physiology (how the body works) and pathology (how the body works in disease) of what is happening. Although you may find certain topics boring (for example, you don't want to be a pathologist, so why should you have to learn how to stare down microscopes?), you must understand the basics before you advance. Remember that the harder you work in your pre-clinical years, the easier it is in your clinical years – and again, the harder you work in your medical degree and the better doctor you become, the easier it will be to get into the specialty of your choice. Keep in mind that if you want to get into the specialty training program after first year residency you will need to distinguish yourself from the other applicants. Participating in medical research with other doctors will add to your CV, indicate that you are interested in research and will network you with a range of doctors. Many doctors love giving their research projects to medical students to complete – so take these opportunities as they arise and don't be afraid to actively seek them out.

Something to keep in mind – all Australian medical students must undergo a placement in a rural setting, during some point of their medical degree. For most this is only 4 to 8 weeks, but for others this may be as long as a year. It is a great opportunity to see different parts of Australia, and will prepare you better as you get to see different things, and may even give you a more hands-on experience. In addition, most medical schools include an 'elective' term, in which you may choose which hospital you wish to do a rotation of study in. Often, this can be anywhere in the world, and is an amazing experience.

'My favourite part of medical school was my elective in Armenia. I had an eye-opening experience and saw first-hand how desperate some regions of the world are. I came to appreciate how fortunate we are in this blessed nation of ours and how important it is for us to safeguard our healthcare system so our children and their children can enjoy the same benefits we have.'

Dr Zorik Avakian, Orthopaedic Registrar

A great resource is the Australian Medical Students Association (AMSA). Their website, www.amsa.org.au contains a range of information for all potential and current (and graduating) medical students, including how to maintain your physical and mental health (www.amsa.org.au/wellbeing) and how to manage anxiety and depression (http://www.amsa.org.au/projects/wellbeing/depression-and-anxiety-what-can-you-do-about-it/).

Something additional I should mention: medical school is one of the last opportunities to enjoy free time. As a doctor you will be working long, unpredictable hours so enjoy your hobbies, friends and freedom while you can!

Pre-clinical Years

If you have completed an undergraduate degree previously, especially a science degree, your pre-clinical years will be nothing new. However, if you have come straight from high school, university will be a whole new experience – no one is taking the roll to make sure you're at class and no one will spoon-feed you the information, so you need to keep up your hard work!

Something new, even for those who have already completed an undergraduate degree are 'PBLs'. The pre-clinical years of medicine are based on a style of learning called problem-based learning (PBL) which was developed in Canada in the 1960s, and since then many medical schools (and even some business and engineering schools) have adopted this approach.

As such, you no longer study one subject called anatomy and another subject called pathology, but instead you utilise problem-based learning, in which you have a case that you focus on, and learn all the medical sciences relevant to that case. For example, if the PBL is focusing on lung cancer, that week your lectures and tutorials will focus on areas such as the anatomy of the lungs, the physiology of respiration and gas exchange, the pathophysiology of lung cancer, as well as a lecture on the effects of smoking, and public health policies to reduce smoking in the community (just to name a few). This way, you are not learning disjointed parts of information that don't fit clearly together (imagine studying the anatomy of the foot, while learning about the physiology of the heart, while learning about the embryology of the head and neck – it would be incredibly confusing!), but instead your learning is based on a central problem which allows you to have a coherent understanding where everything fits together.

PBLs (the tutorials themselves) are more expensive for the university and demand more time from both the students and the academic staff, but they work, making graduates feel more prepared (Dean 2003), and producing better medical students and doctors (Koh 2008, Smits 2002). It teaches you not just about medicine, but about how to research information, work in a team and solve a problem.

'Medicine is endless and it is easy to get bogged down in detail. Go for breadth over depth. Make sure that no area is neglected but the sooner you realise that you don't need the minute details the easier life will become for you.'

Dr Ed Campion, Intern, St Vincent's Hospital Sydney

An important note for medical school study – often notes from the previous year are available from other students for you to use. Many students use these as their only study notes, or sometimes will print them out and make additional notes on them. This may get you through your degree, but will not get you good marks, or make you a good doctor. A 2006 study demonstrated that 'students who create their own study aids are spending time making them, whereas those who use others' study aids are not. It may also be that the process of creating study aids helps the learner gain more meaningful knowledge through the process of synthesizing disparate pieces of information into new knowledge' (Sleight 2006). So do your own study, and don't rely on notes from others!

One last study tip – make yourself a 'To do' list at the beginning of each week. This allows you to prioritise your work, and tick off each item as you complete it.

Anatomy

Anatomy deals with the study of the structure of the human body. This is one of the most difficult topics for many medical students, as it is incredibly complex and very detailed. I am afraid the only way to learn anatomy is to expose yourself to the content over and over again.

Start with a basic anatomy textbook (for example Anatomedia, or an anatomy colouring book such as that by Kaplan 2009 – see the References section) to give you a simple overview of the basics of anatomy. Move onto a clinical anatomy textbook (some are listed below) and work through it from the beginning, complementing this with the Acland's DVD set (see the Further Reading section in the back of this book).

Read the relevant chapters before your anatomy labs and refer to your pre-made notes while looking at the dissected specimens. This helps consolidate the textbook knowledge with what the human body actually looks like.

Anatomy is a great subject for mnemonics (see Chapter 3: 'Study Techniques' for more on mnemonics). One of the most famous medical student mnemonics is that for the carpal bones of the hand: 'Some lovers try positions that they can't handle', standing for scaphoid, lunate, triquetral, pisiform, trapezium, trapezoid, capitate and hamate. There are many books (including Kahn 2008 – see the References section) full of mnemonics, but none stick better in your mind than those you make up yourself.

Biochemistry and Physiology

Physiology is the study of the function of the human body while biochemistry deals with the function of the human body on a molecular level, and thus physiology and biochemistry are undoubtedly intertwined.

For those that struggle with physiology, start with a combined anatomy-physiology textbook (for example, Marieb 2012) for a quick overview. Alternatively, start right in with Guyton and Hall's *Textbook of Medical Physiology*, which details biochemistry and physiology (see the References section for these books).

No part of biochemistry or physiology can be neglected. That is, you must understand function on a cellular level as well as a tissue and system level for complete understanding. There is no point understanding that a lack of blood supply to the brain is deleterious unless you can understand how crucial oxygen is to generation of ATP via aerobic respiration.

Pharmacology

Pharmacology deals with the study of drugs and how they interact with the human body in health and disease. A good pharmacology textbook will cover the physiology, pathophysiology and pharmacology (for example, Rang 2011), so is a great subject for consolidating your knowledge.

Summarising information into tables is helpful, and especially great for pharmacology. For example, if summarising the pharmacology of statins, this may look something like:

Drug Type	Action	Side Effects	Examples
Statin	Inhibit HMG-CoA Reductase (catalyses conversion of HMG-CoA to mevalonic acid) = ↓ cholesterol synthesis = ↓ TGs, LDL & total cholesterol, & ↑ HDL	Myalgia/myositis, rhabdomyolysis, altered LFTs	Atorvastatin (Lipitor), rosuvastatin (Crestor), simvastatin (Zocor), pravastatin (Lipostat)

Do not be concerned with drug doses until you are in your final year. Once you are in the hospital every day, being exposed to drug doses on a regular basis will allow it to sink in via osmosis (helped by a bit of reading). However, a great book that includes doses, routes, pharmacokinetics, drug interactions, indications, contraindications and side effects and thus is great for your clinical years is *Drugs in Anaesthesia and Intensive Care*, 4th edition (see the References section).

Pathophysiology

Pathophysiology deals with the study of the human body in disease. Many students struggle with this, especially on a cellular level, as the textbooks often go into detail on abnormal mitoses, fragmented cytoplasm, speckled chromatin and more. Don't worry too much about the detail, just achieve a general understanding of the disease process on a cellular, tissue and system level, and leave the exquisite detail to the pathologists.

Like all of medicine, spend some time looking at pictures of *normal* tissues, so you can tell when something is abnormal. For example, if you know what normal lung tissue looks like under a microscope, you know that something is wrong when you see a slide of an emphysematous lung, or a bronchial carcinoma.

Microbiology

Microbiology is the study of microorganisms, and how they interact with the human body.

Do not worry if you can't remember all of the microbes' names, or which ones are Gram-negative rods, which agar plates certain microbes grow on, or which antibiotic kills which bacteria. Like most of medicine, you will pick up the clinically relevant information with repeat exposure. In fact, most clinicians just remember a few antibiotics which will cover a broad range of organisms and use those repeatedly.

Aim to understand which microorganisms usually live in each part of the body, which pathogens usually invade each part of the body and which antibiotic you can use on each – this will be more than enough understanding for any medical student!

Diseases

A great study tip for medical school (and even physicians or surgical training) is organising each disease under subheadings of:

- Epidemiology – how many people are affected, and whether males or females, or people of certain ethnicities are more at risk
- Aetiology – the cause(s) of the disease
- Pathophysiology – what happens on a cellular or tissue level

- <u>Presentation</u> – what symptoms and signs the patients will present with
- <u>Investigations</u> – what tests you might like to order
- <u>Diagnosis and/or classification</u> – the requirements for diagnosis, or how the different sub-types of the disease are classified
- <u>Treatment</u> – what management (social, medical and surgical) is needed
- <u>Prognosis</u> – the survival rate, and rate of complications

This covers 99 percent of everything you need to know about each condition, and is a great resource to have for quick revision. This is especially good to summarise into tables, which may look like, see for example on next page.

For more on methods to study effectively at university, refer to Chapter 3: 'Study Techniques'.

'Study with friends. As everyone is in a different hospital each of you will have different tips and tricks for clinical exams, as well as deeper information on different topics. This is also more relaxing and reaffirming than studying alone.

Write palm cards for specific points that you find hard to remember and keep them with you – go over them whilst on the bus, or give them to a family member/friend/boyfriend/girlfriend and get them to quiz you.'

Emily Sutherland, High Distinction Student, Sixth Year Medicine, University of New South Wales

---

'Have organised notes so that when exam time comes at the end of the year you have a system for reviewing them.'

Anika Johnston, High Distinction Student, Sixth Year Medicine, University of New South Wales

---

'Studying medicine is different from high school in that most of it is "self-directed". This makes it even more crucial to work hard consistently throughout the year. There is a wide variety of resources available for studying and this should definitely be utilised. Study groups make a significant contribution to the process and allow the individual to discuss concerns with colleagues as well as gauge how well they are progressing relative to others.'

Dr Zorik Avakian, Orthopaedic Registrar

Disease	Epidemiology	Aetiology	Pathophysiology	Presentation	Investigations	Diagnosis and Classification	Treatment	Prognosis
Heart Failure (HF)	1.5–2% pop., >50% pts >85 years	Ischemic heart disease and hypertension (mostly), diabetes, pulmonary hypertension, outflow obstruction, arrhythmias	↓ cardiac contractility (or dilatation) → ↓ejection fraction → ↓cardiac output (CO), causing stimulation of RAAS → vasoconstriction, Na^+ and H_2O retention, and SNS activation → supports CO initially, but eventually causes fluid overload → pulmonary and peripheral oedema	Low CO = fatigue, cold peripheries, hypotension and oliguria Left HF = mildly raised JVP, pulmonary oedema (dyspnoea, paroxysmal nocturnal dyspnoea, inspiratory creps), pleural effusion, cardiomegaly, and mild pitting oedema Right HF = high JVP, hepatic and splenic congestion, peripheral oedema and ascites	FBC, EUC, Hb, TFTs, BG, ECG, CXR, BNP, Echo	Largely clinical Dx	1) ACE-inhibitor/ Sartan + beta-blocker + spironolactone 2) Diuretics (for euvolemia) 3) Digoxin (for symptom relief or AF) 4) Consider antiarrhythmics and anticoagulation	NYHA I – 5% annual mortality NYHA II – 10% NYHA IV – 40–60%

Clinical Years

Congratulations on making it this far – this is where the real fun begins! In your clinical years you will be on rotations in hospitals – watching and helping in surgeries, taking blood, cannulating and catheterising patients, being in the hospital learning and observing until the early hours of the morning... what you've always dreamed about! This is when you start to feel like a real doctor.

> *'Medicine cannot be learnt entirely from textbooks and lectures. Whilst these are obviously important, it is time with patients that will cement your learning and make you remember that x set of symptoms equals y condition.'*
>
> Anika Johnston, High Distinction Student, Sixth Year Medicine, University of New South Wales

You are likely to be doing 4- to 8-week placements rotating through different specialties (different surgical specialties, internal medicine, emergency, psychiatry, obstetrics and gynecology, anaesthetics, general practice and so on), getting as much hands on experience as you can. Some rotations will only be for a few hours a day in which you are expected to be at the hospital. Some students take this as an opportunity to do as little as possible, only showing up for teaching rounds. However, other students will take this as an opportunity to show their dedication and willingness to learn by staying with their allocated medical team and participating/helping where possible. Often staying on at the hospital at night will ensure you more opportunities for hands on work as there are less staff on duty, and sometimes the most interesting cases arrive at night!

When entering a new hospital or work place, treat the staff and other health professionals with respect. You, as a medical student, are a visitor to their workplace and must be respectful to each individual's role. Nurses can be of great assistance to medical students, so respect them and they will teach you and give you plenty of help and guidance. When I placed my first cannula, it was a nurse who supervised me and passed me the bung that I had forgotten to prepare, and so saved me from having the patient bleed all over the bed. Disrespect nurses, and your clinical years will be not only limited, but also a nightmare!

'Go through each topic you cover as soon as you can, but also try to relate each topic back to your hospital time. Try to find specific patients who have pathologies you have recently learnt about in lectures as this way you can truly understand how the pathology manifests as a clinical presentation.'

Emily Sutherland, High Distinction Student, Sixth Year Medicine, University of New South Wales

Some days will be tiring. Starting at the hospital at 7am and finishing at 7 or even 10pm, you then have to go home to start studying… Or, you have been in the emergency department until 3am and have to be at university for lectures at 8am… Doesn't sound like fun does it? Well you are wrong! It is the most amazing fun, and you will not regret a second of it. Sometimes you will be in the hospital overnight, whether you are staying to watch a birth, or because you were extra keen and told the registrar that if an interesting surgery comes in overnight (or over the weekend), they should call you and you will come right in. However, it is draining, and you must have a hobby or interests outside university and the hospital, or you won't survive the intensity of medical school.

Another piece of advice – never underestimate the importance of sleep! When I was getting 4 hours of sleep every night in order to fit in exercise, hospital time and study, my marks dropped – even though I was doing twice as much study as the year before. You need sleep, not just to survive (I know many medical students – myself included – that think they can sleep when they graduate), but for your brain to function most effectively, and learn as much as possible.

Balancing clinical time and time spent in the books is difficult. You may need to begin studying on weekends (if you are not already) in order to get your weekly reading done, or just be really efficient during the week! However, it is crucial that you don't miss out on interesting cases in the hospital just to go home and study – you will be assessed partly on your clinical skills and partly on your knowledge of the basic clinical sciences, so make sure you balance these two (easier said than done).

Q: What was your favourite part of medical school?

A: *The last 2 years of the course. The pre-clinical 'theory' years finally made some sense. Integrating the theory with the practice of medicine actually takes some years as a postgraduate to achieve.*

Associate Professor Andrew Dean, Consultant Emergency Physician, St John of God Hospital, Ballarat

Presenting a Patient

In general, presenting patients to colleagues follows a set pattern:

- <u>Name, age and sex</u> – Consider also adding their occupation (for example, if you suspect their occupation as a baker is worsening their asthma), or their current social situation (for example, if the patient is now dependent on others due to an acute deterioration in function) if relevant.

- <u>Presenting complaint</u> – The reason for presentation and the duration of the complaint. This may be 'the patient has a 3-hour history of central crushing chest pain' (the symptom), or 'the patient presented for a left total hip replacement' (the procedure), depending on the situation.

- <u>History of presenting complaint</u> – Characterise the presenting complaint, outline pertinent negatives and other symptoms associated with the presenting complaint (for example, if the patient presents short of breath, also mention the fact that they have a productive cough and a fever).

- <u>Past medical history</u> – Discuss past medical and surgical history, and any complications.

- <u>Medications</u> – Drugs, doses, route and frequency.

- <u>Allergies</u> – Not just what they are allergic too, but what happens when exposed to that allergen. There is a big difference between feeling nauseous when given morphine, and suffering anaphylaxis when given penicillin.

- <u>Social history</u> – Occupational status, and whether they are independent in their activities of daily living (if relevant).

- <u>Smoking, alcohol and drug use</u> – Quantified.

- <u>Family history</u> – Immediate family members.

- <u>Systems review</u> – Relevant to the current presentation.

- <u>Examination findings</u> – Relevant to the presenting complaint. For example, do not mention the patient's total knee replacement scar in a suspected myocardial infarct.

- <u>Summary</u> – Summarise the information in one or two sentences. For example, 'In summary, John Smith is a 68-year-old who presented this morning with acute onset crushing central chest pain and dyspnoea, on a background of ischaemic heart disease.'

- <u>Your differential diagnosis</u> – List your differential in order of likelihood. For example, 'He is likely suffering an acute coronary syndrome, but possible differentials include unstable angina and pulmonary embolus.'

- <u>Investigation plan</u> – List investigations in order that you think they should be done, namely in terms of ease and expense. For example, if you think your patient has suffered a cerebrovascular event, list your investigations in the order: ECG, blood glucose, blood lipids, FBC, UEC, coagulation screen, then non-contrast CT.

- <u>Management plan</u> – If the investigation results are already back or you would like to start empirical therapy (for example, in the case of suspected pneumonia or an acute coronary syndrome), briefly outline your management plan in chronological order. Consider mentioning any issues outstanding (for example, the patient may need to see an ophthalmologist to have their eyes checked for diabetic complications, a consult with a dietician for management of their obesity and an aged-care-assessment team to ascertain whether the patient needs extra help at home).

Although you may take a more detailed history than the one you present to your clinician, tailor your presentation to the clinical situation and the clinician (see below). (A good paper on how to present a clinical case is by Olaitan 2010, see the References section.)

Presenting a patient differs depending on the situation (whether a formal presentation, or a quick overview of the patient), and what specialty you are currently in. For example:

- <u>Internal medicine</u> – A physician will want a thorough, detailed medical history and examination, containing all relevant positives and negatives. There is no such thing as too much detail when presenting to a physician.

- <u>Surgery</u> – Your surgeon will want a detailed history and a thorough physical examination, with a special focus on potential peri-operative complications; such as anti-coagulation, diabetes, or cervical spine instability (regardless of surgical specialty).

- <u>Emergency</u> – Emergency physicians have no time for drawn out, detailed presentations. You need to grab their attention in the first sentence, and ideally get the whole case presented in under 60 seconds – just pretend you've called a consultant at 3am, and need to present the case before they fall back asleep. For example 'John Smith is a 68-year-old retired accountant who this morning suffered acute onset of crushing central chest pain and dyspnoea, on a background of worsening angina over two weeks. He is a vasculopath with two previous stents in 2006 and a coronary bypass graft in 2008, hypertension, type 2 diabetes, hyperlipidemia, and a 50-pack-year smoking history. He is currently tachycardic at 110, hypotensive to 90/40, saturating at 88 percent on 10 litres via Hudson mask. My main concern is an acute coronary syndrome, so I would like to insert a cannula, order a FBC, UEC, troponin, blood glucose, ECG and chest X-ray, and give pain relief, aspirin and clopidogrel pending the results of the ECG and troponin.' (A great paper for presenting cases in the emergency department is by Davenport 2008, see the References section.)

On the Wards

The wards are a great opportunity to put into practice everything you have spent the past few years learning from textbooks and lectures. If you are keen to learn about how heart failure presents, head up to the cardiac ward. If you have a presentation on liver failure, the gastro ward. You can often use the hospital computer system to search for patients with individual diagnoses, if you are looking to learn about a particular disease. Alternatively, just head to the right ward and ask the nurses if they have any interesting patients, or any patients that are friendly and wouldn't mind having a chat with you. However, don't overwhelm the patient by turning up with a group of medical students – limit it to you and (if you must) one other medical student. Remember that the patients are ill, and aren't there to be your teaching resource. Also, remember to always respect patient confidentiality!

A good idea is to print out the patient list of the team that you are with. This way, you know the patient names and locations, can write what you need to do (for example, if you have been asked to take a FBC and UEC from a patient, under the patients name write: ☐ 'FBC/UEC' so you can tick off the box once you have done this), can remind yourself to chase the results of any tests, and so on.

Be interested and helpful. If you show that you are keen to learn, the staff will be keen to teach. Remember that you are there as an observer, and the staff are often not being paid (or not being paid very much) to look after you – so don't get in their way, or be a nuisance. In fact, if you offer to help (whether clerking patients, inserting cannulas, or helping nurses mobilise patients to the bathroom) you will not only learn, but also assist the ward staff who will be grateful. If asked to perform a procedure you have never done before and you feel uncomfortable, be honest with the doctor or nurse. They will either do it themselves with you observing, or assist you and talk you through it.

A new skill you must acquire on the wards is answering questions posed by the clinicians. It is important that you have a good system for answering difficult questions, because even if you do not know the correct answer, they will still be impressed if you demonstrate good, logical reasoning. For example, if after examining a patient you are asked the cause of a patient's epigastric pain, you are not expected to give a definitive diagnosis (e.g., 'acute pancreatitis secondary to azathioprine use') right away. It is reasonable (and possibly more impressive) if you can give an answer like 'The patient's epigastric pain radiates to the back, so is probably due to acute pancreatitis. The patient is febrile, but a negative Murphy's sign makes cholecystitis less likely, and a lack of relation to meals makes peptic ulcer disease less likely.' Thinking aloud allows the clinician to see your reasoning, and even if you are wrong, it demonstrates that you understand the problem and are working through it in a reasonable, logical manner.

In addition, do not answer their questions with a question. Be decisive, even if you are unsure. For example, if asked where the uterine artery originates, do not answer 'Is it the internal iliac artery?' This makes you seem unsure, so even if you are correct, they are less likely to think you have any knowledge at all. Instead, just say 'The uterine artery originates from the internal iliac artery'. This makes you seem confident, so even if your answer is incorrect, it seems like an honest mistake, rather than you guessing randomly. Answering in full sentences also makes your knowledge more coherent.

It is also likely that you will get questions wrong, but don't let it get to you. I get embarrassed when I answer a question incorrectly, so I make sure I never forget the answer – so getting questions wrong is actually a great learning experience!

It seems obvious, but dress and act as you would expect a doctor treating one of your family members – that is, helpful, caring, polite and professional.

Important advice – always check with the nurses before you see their patient. Even if the consultant has asked you to see one of their patients, ask the nurse on the ward if that is OK with them. They may be about to do a set of obs (observations, taking the patients vital signs), give medications or perform pressure-area care, and will tell you to come back later. Otherwise, they will be more than happy for you to speak to their patient, and showing them courtesy is extremely important – and gets you into good habits for later life, as no-one likes an arrogant medical student or doctor.

When you are in your final years, act like an intern. Assess your patient and write up comprehensive notes in the file (in the SOAP format – see 'Ward Rounds' below), including what you think is happening with the patient (their diagnosis or their progress), investigations you would like (to confirm your diagnosis and exclude differential diagnoses) and your proposed treatment plan. Compare your management plan with what the team implements, to see if you are on the right track.

Ward Rounds

Ward rounds (when the treating team sees each of their patients every morning) are an important part of your clinical day. Tips include:

- Know each of your patients, including:
  - Their name
  - Why they've been admitted to hospital
  - How long they have been in hospital
  - What are the significant results of their investigations, surgeries etc.
- If possible, get to hospital early and review each of your patients *before* rounds, especially what has changed since yesterday, including:
  - Vitals
  - Investigation results
  - Pain scores
- Importantly, *speak* to your patients before you round with your team. Find out:
  - How they are feeling in general
  - How they slept
  - What their pain levels are like
  - If anything has changed
  - If they have any concerns
- Show that you are interested. Ask questions and offer to help at any opportunity.
- Offer to scribe (write in the notes while the consultant, registrar or resident assesses the patient). A good format is the SOAP format (subjective, objective, assessment and plan), which includes:
  - The date and time
  - The team currently assessing the patient
  - Your name and role (medical student), and the team assessing the patient
  - How the patient feels (Subjective) – e.g., how they are feeling, their level of pain

- ○ What the physical examination, and results from blood tests and other investigations showed (Objective)

- ○ What the team thinks the differential diagnosis is, or how the patient is progressing (Assessment)

- ○ What the Management Plan is, and when each part of the plan is to be completed

- ○ Your signature, and the counter-signature of one of the doctors

- Have pathology or radiology request forms, or discharge summary sheets with you at all times – consultants will be impressed if you can provide them with the form they need on the spot.

Not only will these habits be great preparation for internship, but will also set you well above most of the other medical students (even other interns and residents) in the eyes of your consultant, and improve your accessibility to registrar/consultant teaching and extra-curricular opportunities (for example, theatre time in interesting cases) and your marks at the end of your rotation.

Theatre

In the theatre, there will probably be the following staff:

- Head surgeon (usually a consultant surgeon, but may be a surgical registrar)

- Assisting surgeon (this may be another consultant surgeon or a surgical registrar)

- Scrub nurse (a nurse who is scrubbed for theatre and helps the surgeon with his or her equipment)

- Scout nurse (a nurse who is not scrubbed and therefore is able to get more equipment if needed, and counts the surgical equipment)

- Anaesthetist

- Anaesthetic nurse

Infection is the most feared complication of surgery, and as a result the surgical staff take infection control very seriously. Abide by all infection-control policies and you will have no trouble. To do this (and other tips for theatre, including for how to get on-side with theatre staff), suggestions include:

- Introduce yourself to all the theatre staff (listed above) before the list starts

- Wear a mask at all times once the sterile equipment has been opened

- Don't touch the sterile area if you are not scrubbed (even take care walking near sterile areas)

- Ask one of the nurses where they would like you to stand

- Don't stand between the anaesthetist and the anaesthetic trolley or monitoring equipment

- If scrubbing in for theatre:

  ○ Tell the theatre nurses that you've been asked to scrub

  ○ Offer to get your own gloves and gown (so the nurse does not have to do it for you)

  ○ Start scrubbing before your consultant does

- Don't touch the scrub nurse's surgical tray (whether you are scrubbed or not)

- Don't speak to the surgeons or nurses if they are acutely focused on something

- Help in transferring patients to and from the theatre trolley

- As always, be honest if you don't know what to do – everyone will be more than happy to help you out

If you know you will be watching an operation the next day, make sure that you read the anatomy and the steps of the procedure itself before walking into the theatre (this is often freely available on the internet). Not only will you get more out of the experience, you will also impress the surgeon!

The Emergency Department

The ED is a great place to get hands on experience, and finally feel like 'a real doctor'. You will often be allowed to see patients before other doctors have, and perform procedures like cannulating, suturing and assorted other activities (for example, retrieving foreign bodies like buttons or erasers that children have inserted into their nose). As ED is often very busy, doctors will often encourage you to assess patients (taking a history and performing a physical examination), and then ask what investigations *you* would like to order, and what *your* initial management plan is. This is fantastic experience! If you let the nurses know you are keen to help, they will often get you to insert cannulas or take blood.

Often you do not need to wait until your ED rotation – just find a doctor who is happy to have you around, and make yourself known. Once you become a familiar face, the staff will not only be happy to have you, but will often come and get you if there is an interesting case, or something fun for you to do! See the 'Student's Guide to the Emergency Department' in Gordian Fulde's Book *Emergency Medicine: The Principles of Practice*, 6th edition, for more tips on surviving in the emergency department.

> **Q:** What is one piece of advice you would like to pass on to aspiring medical students?
>
> **A:** *Never forget why they wanted to do medicine in the first place, as we often forget this and without realising it, become the very doctor we said we would never be!!*
>
> *One important tip – always remember to treat every patient as you would your own family!!!*
>
> Dr Zorik Avakian, Orthopaedic Registrar

Radiology

Radiology is a tough area for medical students, and the only way to learn is practice. It helps to have a system for interpreting medical imaging, especially when you are starting out. You may like to invent your own system, but I have outlined some approaches you can take to interpreting chest and abdominal radiographs (X-rays).

<u>All imaging</u> – Start interpretation of all imaging by assessing the following:

- Ensure you have the right patient (by checking name, age and sex)
- The date the image was taken
- Whether the radiograph was erect, supine or decubitus
- If a side-marker is present
- If the patient is rotated
- If there is sufficient penetration (for a chest radiograph, you should just be able to make out the lower thoracic vertebral bodies through the heart)
- If there is sufficient inspiration for a chest radiograph (on an erect X-ray, the diaphragm should be at the level of the 6th rib anteriorly, or the 10th rib posteriorly)

Chest radiograph – Remember this with 'ABCDEFGH':

A. AIRWAY – the trachea should be central and non-obstructed.

B. BONES and SOFT TISSUE – any fractures, lytic or sclerotic lesions, or soft tissue pathology. Also check for presence of breast shadows.

C. CARDIAC SHADOW – you should be able to identify the left atrium and ventricle and the right atrium, and the heart should takes up less than 50 percent of the thoracic diameter.

D. DIAPHRAGM – surfaces should be convex, with the right hemidiaphragm higher than the left, and no fluid in the costophrenic angles.

E. EQUAL LUNG VOLUMES – count the ribs on each side, looking for hyperinflation or collapse/consolidation.

F. FINE DETAIL and FOREIGN BODIES – observe the lung parenchyma (excluding pneumothoracies, masses, consolidation or collapse) and vasculature of the lungs (excluding dilated pulmonary vasculature).

G. GAS – look for the gastric bubble and for gas under the diaphragm.

H. HILA – the left hilum should be up to 3cm higher than the right, and enlarged lymph nodes make the hila look bulky.

Abdominal radiograph – Remember this with 'ABCDEF'

A. AIR – normal gas (gastric bubble, gas in bowel) and gas outside viscera (exclude pneumoperitoneum, or air in the biliary tree, bowel wall or portal vein).

B. BONE – assess density, and exclude any fractures, or lytic/sclerotic lesions.

C. CALCIFICATION – of soft tissues and blood vessels.

D. DILATATION – of viscera (for example, a bowel obstruction). Remember that small intestine is usually in the centre of the film, is under three centimetres in diameter and has valvulae conniventes which cross the whole bowel diameter. In contrast, the colon is on the periphery of the radiograph (forms a 'window-frame'), is under five centimetres in diameter (the cecum is bigger, but still under nine centimetres), and has haustra which cross only part of the bowel wall.

E. EVIDENT VISCERA – assess the size and shape of any visible soft tissues or organs (for example, the spleen should be 3 ribs long and the kidneys should be 3.5 vertebral bodies long)

F. FLUID LEVELS and FOREIGN BODIES – remember that over five fluid levels is pathological.

> 'Radiology is absolutely fascinating, it's like being in an art gallery every day. It's amazing using images and new technologies to interface with diseases and health, and to support preventative care. It allows you to work with so many fantastic and interesting people and to interact on so many different levels.'
>
> Professor Suzanne Anderson, Consultant Radiologist, Southern Health Radiology, Melbourne

Recommended Textbooks

I recommend you purchase the textbooks suggested by your university, as these books often cover exactly the content your medical school wants you to learn. For some medical students these textbooks do not suit their learning needs (i.e., there is too much or not enough detail, or there is a lack of pictures and diagrams etc.). Even if you choose the most basic book and learn it back-to-front, you will know twice as much as someone who has the most detailed book, but only knows 5 percent of its content.

Popular medical books include:

- *Davidson's Principles and Practice of Medicine*: A great textbook to carry you through medical school, used by most universities. Well explained, great diagrams, and a great variety of information, currently in its 21st edition. Written for use in the UK.

- *Kumar and Clark's Clinical Medicine*: Similar to Davidson's, this is a great book that contains well explained, well-illustrated information, and is currently in its 7th edition. Written for use in the UK.

- *Harrison's Principles of Internal Medicine*: Expensive and contains almost 3,000 pages of detailed information, but has everything you ever wanted to know about every topic. Currently in its 18th edition. Written for use in the United States.

- *The Oxford Handbook of Clinical Medicine*: Not a big thick medical 'textbook' (more of a pocket book), but contains well referenced, well explained, current information on most diseases known to man – a medical student favourite (especially as it is a perfect size to carry around on the wards). Currently in its 8th edition, and written for use in the UK.

- *Emergency Medicine: The Principles of Practice*: As the title suggests, a book on emergency medicine written by Australia's leading emergency physician (Professor Gordian Fulde, Director of Accident and Emergency at St Vincent's Hospital, Sydney). Covers all possible emergency medicine scenarios, which are all well explained, with easily found emergency flow charts and drug doses. Currently in its 6th edition, and written for use in Australia.

- *Clinical Examination* (commonly known as 'Talley and O'Connor'): A textbook on how to take histories and conduct physical examinations, standard reading at most medical schools. Currently in its 6th edition, it is written for use in Australia.

- *Davidson's Principles and Practice of Surgery*: A surgical textbook which covers the basics of the principles of surgery. Currently in its 5th edition, written for use in the UK.

> 'Get into a good routine early in your course and be consistent. I was part of a study group from first year and I found it really helpful. Be organised.'
>
> Dr Catherine Crane, Senior Resident, Concord Hospital, Sydney

> 'Realise that you need to nurture your body as well as your mind, so attend practical sessions in fresh air, ensure you exercise and maintain social contact with non-medical friends throughout your studies.'
>
> Associate Professor Andrew Dean, Consultant Emergency Physician, St John of God Hospital, Ballarat

Popular medical science books include:

- *Robbins and Cotran: Pathologic Basis of Disease:* An incredibly detailed, yet well explained and illustrated pathology textbook, currently in its 8th edition. Standard reading at most medical schools.

- *Clinically Oriented Anatomy* or *Gray's Anatomy for Students*: Both are excellent anatomy textbooks in their 6th and 2nd editions respectively, with added clinical information that makes it easy to remember and relevant to the practice of medicine. All medical students should have a good anatomy textbook! You might also like to skip straight to *Last's Anatomy: Regional and Applied*, 12th edition, the prescribed anatomy text for the Australasian College of Surgeons.

- *Guyton and Hall Textbook of Medical Physiology:* A great physiology textbook used by science and medical students for years, written in a very conversational manner, with great explanations, diagrams and pictures. Currently in its 12th edition, and one of my personal favourites.

- *Rang and Dale's Pharmacology*: Incredibly well explained and illustrated pharmacology book, used by both medical students and pharmacology majors. Currently in its 7th edition, it covers the relevant pharmacology, physiology and pathology.

In addition there are many DVDs to help you learn. For example Acland's is a DVD which teaches very detailed anatomy in a very easy-to-understand way.

Backing Up Work

One last tip that is crucial – back up your work. If you have anything stored on your computer or USB, store a copy somewhere else. I thought I was pretty good at backing up my work (I would save files from my USB to my computer every couple of weeks), but once left my USB in the pocket of a pair of scrubs, and lost 2 weeks worth of study notes. It wasn't fun trying to keep up with my weekly study, as well as re-doing the notes that I had lost! Another horror story comes from my best friend, who had his only copy of his honours research on his laptop which was stolen from his car, and so had to re-do his entire research and thesis.

Get into a good habit early on by regularly backing-up onto an external hard drive, a USB, to your laptop, or sending important files to an email account that you use only for backing up. Just make sure you have some kind of system to save your information – there is enough study without having to do it twice!

> **Q:** What are your tips for studying in medical school?
>
> **A:** *Go to lectures, don't get too far behind, and keep up your sports, hobbies and social life.*
>
> Dr Elspeth Fotheringham, General Practitioner, Tuggerah

> *'Study together with other med students – it makes it so much less boring and testing each other's knowledge is really helpful.'*
>
> Anika Johnston, High Distinction Student, Sixth Year Medicine, University of New South Wales

Finances, Accommodation and Transport

Finances

Funding a medical degree is challenging at the best of times, but this becomes especially difficult if you have a full-fee-paying place. Commonwealth Supported Places cost around $9,000; while full-fee-paying places can cost between $25,000 and $50,000. Thankfully, you can defer your payment until you graduate (see Chapter 8: 'The Application' for details).

However, you still must fund your textbooks and other expenses, and if you live out of home, pay rent and eat! Fitting a part-time job around your busy academic schedule is difficult, and something many students struggle with. I was lucky enough to find a job which allowed me to work in a hospital environment on the weekends, with spare time which allowed me to study while at work. Many of my colleagues worked as nurses or orderlies at local hospitals. However, many students find work in cafes, department stores, bars, pharmacies and a variety of places. The important thing is not allowing your paid work to impact your study, due to working long hours, working during the week, or just working too hard that you cannot focus on your study.

Remember that life isn't only about work and study – it is OK to have time to relax and enjoy life!

Many universities offer scholarships in various forms. These include research scholarships and academic scholarships – and don't be afraid to apply. I wrote one successful application for a research scholarship in an internet cafe whilst travelling in Munich, so you have to be in it to win it!

Scholarships outside of your university include:

- John Flynn Placement Program – successful students complete two-week placements in the same rural or remote community for four years, and receive $500 per week for the two weeks, plus the cost of travel and accommodation. 300 students are selected each year. See www.acrrm.org.au/about-john-flynn-placement-program for more information.

- Rural Australia Medical Undergraduate Scholarship – the Australian Government selects 120 students with a rural background and demonstrated financial need each year, to receive $10,000 annually throughout their degree. See http://ramus.ruralhealth.org.au/ for more information.

- Puggy Hunter Memorial Scholarship – the Australian Government offers Aboriginal and Torres Strait Islander students $15,000 per year during their medical degree if selected to receive this scholarship. See www.rcna.org.au/

WCM/RCNA/Scholarships/Government/puggy_hunter/rcna/scholarships/
government/puggy_hunter_memorial_scholarship_scheme.aspx for more
information.

* Defence Force Scholarship – the Australian Defence Force (ADF) offers
  undergraduates (who have already completed one year of a three or four
  year degree or two years of a five or six year degree) $43,266, and graduates
  $64,437 per year as a salary during your degree. Students also have their
  university fees paid, and receive free healthcare, subsidised accommodation,
  and a textbook allowance. In return, once you graduate you must work for
  the ADF for the number of years you received the scholarship, plus one
  (that is, you will be an army or navy doctor for however many years they
  paid for your degree, plus one). See www.defencejobs.gov.au/education/
  universitysponsorship/ for more details.

Loans are another viable source of income for medical students. If you can't
convince your parents to give you an interest free loan, many banks offer
student loans – although the interest is often over 10 percent per year, and
some banks require you to have a part time job before they will give you the
loan. One company does offer loans purely for medical students with interest
rates less than that of the banks, as well as only requiring you to pay back your
loan once you graduate – see www.promedfinance.com.au for more details.
Your university will also have more information on student loans.

Accommodation and Transport

Many students have to relocate to attend their chosen medical school. Your
university will often have student accommodation on offer, or will have a
housing service which will assist you in finding accommodation. Other sources
of rented accommodation include online websites like www.domain.com.
au. Importantly, many students will be in the same situation as you (looking
for cheap accommodation), so organise to share a house with other medical
students. This is not easy if you haven't started university yet, so join the
medical school's Facebook page or attend events for future medical students
to meet others searching for shared accommodation.

The question of transport is an important one in medical school. You may live
close to your universities teaching hospital, but keep in mind you will be sent
all around the city (and even the country) during your medical degree and so
will need good transportation. Even if you forget about the fact that you will
almost certainly be doing a rural rotation at some point, it is likely you will be
doing four to eight week rotations in hospitals a fair distance away from your
home. For this reason, it is desirable that you have access to a car. Whether it

is your own car or you can borrow it from a parent or sibling, it will save you hours in travel time – especially as you are likely to be starting and finishing at university and the hospital at strange hours which may not be conducive to catching public transport.

What Now?

A question you will face all throughout your medical degree (and sometimes even before you get into medical school) is 'What *kind* of doctor do you want to be?' This is a difficult question. As a medical student, you will change your mind multiple times as you learn about each specialty, and then as you rotate through each specialty in the hospital you will love certain areas and hate others. As an intern and resident, you will again rotate through the individual specialties but have more of a hands-on role in managing patients, and will get a better idea of what each specialty has to offer, and whether it suits you. Importantly, many training programs allow you to take time off during your registrar training, giving you time to start a family. Some of the specialties are listed in Chapter 1: 'Introduction'.

> **Q:** Why do you like medicine?
>
> **A:** *There is always change, and you can help patients both individually and as groups. With clinical and other research you are part of a greater picture and supporting change and advances. That is hugely exciting.*
>
> Professor Suzanne Anderson, Consultant Radiologist, Southern Health Radiology

To grossly oversimplify, some benefits and drawbacks of the basic specialties are listed below:

- Surgery – surgical training programs are notoriously difficult to be admitted onto (for example, the Royal Australasian College of Surgeons accepts less than ten cardiothoracic trainees onto their program each year in New South Wales). You often spend long hours in the hospital (as surgeries never keep to the timetable and emergencies always pop up), and may be on call (liable to be called to come into the hospital) more often than not – including in the middle of an anniversary dinner or your son's soccer finals. However, surgery is extremely rewarding. While physicians prescribe medications which may take weeks or months to take effect, you are often able to fix the patients disease immediately. Surgery suits visual, hands-on people with lots of stamina and dedication. See www.surgeons.org for more information, especially their 'Becoming a Surgeon' pages at www.surgeons.org/becoming-a-surgeon/surgery-as-a-career.aspx.

- Internal medicine – internal medicine (practiced by physicians) is thought of as the cerebral specialty, as you aren't using your hands to physically fix someone, but instead are using your knowledge of physiology, pharmacology and pathophysiology to prescribe medications and lifestyle regimens to manage a patient's disease. There are endless specialties (and sub-specialties) for physicians. The lifestyle is less demanding for internal medicine registrars and consultants, but that doesn't mean that training is easy. Often you are able to form long term relationships with your patients and for many, this is one of the best aspects of medicine. See www.racp.edu.au for more information.

- General practice – this is a demanding specialty, requiring the practitioner to be the first port of call for most patients, as well as knowing about all conditions whether medical, surgical or psychiatric, and be able to manage these appropriately. General practice is often chosen due to it facilitating a good work–life balance as you can dictate your own hours, but this depends on the individual practitioner. Another advantage is the ability to practice anywhere in Australia, without the need to establish a referral base (unlike the other specialties). GPs truly build meaningful, long term relationships with patients, and as they are often the first doctor seen by a patient, have a huge amount of trust and respect from their patients. See www.racgp.org.au for more information, especially their 'General Practice Career' pages at www.racgp.org.au/generalpracticecareer.

For a more humorous look at the pros and cons of various specialties, see the book *The House of God* by Samuel Shem (1980). For that matter, all aspiring and current medical students should read *The House of God*, so see 'Medical School Resources' in the back of this book for more information.

Right now, you may be more interested in how much you will be earning as an intern. This differs from state to state, but the base rates (that is, without penalty rates or overtime) in 2012 were:

- NSW $57,422
- ACT $60,186
- NT $63,393

- QLD $65,108
- SA $56,925
- VIC $61,400
- WA $72,295

More information on internship and residency can be found on the AMSA website, www.amsa.org.au/publications/intern-and-residents-guide.

12 | University Information

Below is a list of the medical schools in Australia and New Zealand, classified as undergraduate or postgraduate. Under each medical school is its location, the number and type of places available at time of printing, minimum marks required for entry, average fees (yearly fees for Commonwealth Supported Places, fee for the entire degree for international students) and the medical school website and contact details. Also included below is information on each university from the 'Good Uni Guide' (www.gooduniguide.com.au), including distance from the central business district (CBD), and how students who graduated from that medical school rated their experience compared with average. Cost of nearby accommodation is included (rated from 1 to 5, with 1 described as very low, 2 low, 3 moderate, 4 high and 5 very high). For example, a studio apartment in Kensington (near the University of New South Wales) costs around $350 per week, which earns a rating of 'very high'. Similarly, a studio apartment in Glebe (near Sydney University) costs around $250–300 per week, which earns a rating of 'high'. Each university is ranked according to the Times Higher Education 'World University Rankings 2011– 2012' (www.timeshighereducation.co.uk), both in comparison with other universities in Australia, and also the world. See Chapter 8: 'The Application' for an explanation of the different types of places offered.

All medical schools will require you to pass a 'Working with Children Check' and a 'Police Check', to assure you have no criminal background. Also, you must abide by your state's immunisation policies. Contact your chosen medical school for more information.

A useful source of information on each medical course is the course information sessions held by medical schools throughout the year. Contact your chosen university for more information.

Undergraduate Medical Schools

University of New South Wales

- The UNSW is located in Kensington, Sydney. This is 4km from the CBD, or 15 minutes by bus from Central Station. Cost of living is very high.

- They offer 208 places. These are made up of 96 Commonwealth Supported Places, 52 Bonded Places, 8 Medical Rural Bonded Places, and 52 rural places. They also offer a separate entry stream for Aboriginal and Torres Strait Islander applicants.

- The medical degree is 6 years' duration.

- Rural schools include Albury/Wodonga, Wagga Wagga, Coffs Harbour and Port Macquarie.

- Their main focus is producing excellent doctors, with a focus on research.

- The Kensington campus itself has over 25,000 students, and is one of the most highly regarded medical schools for undergraduates in Australia. In fact, the university itself is ranked 6th in Australia, and 173rd in the world.

- Compared with other Australian medical schools, graduating students rank teaching quality as worse than average, generic skills as worse than average and overall satisfaction as average.

- Average CSP rate is $9,080 per year. Average cost for the degree for international students is $288,000.

- <u>Marks required</u>: UMAT and ATAR marks are interdependent, so the higher your UMAT score the lower ATAR (or equivalent) you need. For example:

  ○ UMAT of 54 per section (raw score) requires an ATAR of 99.95

  ○ UMAT of 70 per section requires an ATAR of 96

- <u>Contact details</u>:

  ○ www.med.unsw.edu.au

  ○ Phone: (02) 9385 8765

  ○ Fax: (02) 9385 1874

  ○ Email: medicine.info@unsw.edu.au

University of Newcastle/University of New England (Joint Medical Program)

- The University of Newcastle is located in Callaghan, Newcastle (10km from the CBD), while the University of New England is located in Armidale (5km from the CBD). Cost of living is low in Callaghan and very low Armidale.

- They offer 170 places, with 110 at the University of Newcastle and 60 at the University of New England. These are made up of 121 Commonwealth Supported Places with 43 Bonded Places and 6 Medical Rural Bonded Places. Thirty percent of these places are offered to applicants with rural or remote backgrounds. They also offer special consideration for Aboriginal and Torres Strait Islander applicants.

- The medical degree is 5 years' duration.
- Rural schools include Taree, Tamworth and Armidale.
- Their main focus is producing excellent doctors, with a focus on producing rural practitioners.
- The Callaghan campus has 20,998 students and the university itself ranks reasonably well academically. In fact, it is ranked 11th in Australia, and 276–300 in the world. The Armidale campus has 3,396 students and ranks reasonably well.
- Comparisons with other Australian medical schools are not available.
- Average CSP rate is $9,080 per year. Average cost of the degree for international students is $187,200.
- Marks required:
  - ATAR: 94.3
  - UMAT of 50 per section
- Contact details:
  - www.newcastle.edu.au/jmp
  - Phone: (02) 4921 5000
  - Fax: (02) 4921 2020
  - Email: enquirycentre@newcastle.edu.au

University of Western Sydney

- The University of Western Sydney's medical school is located in Campbelltown, Sydney. This is 51km from the CBD, and thus cost of accommodation is low.
- They offer 100 Commonwealth Supported Places, with 25 percent of these places for graduate entry.
- The medical degree is 5 years' duration.
- Rural schools include Bathurst and Lismore.
- Their main focus is producing excellent doctors to work in the Greater West.
- The Campbelltown campus has 4,448 students, and the university itself ranks reasonably well academically. It is not part of the Australian or world ranking system.

- Comparisons with other Australian medical schools are not available.

- Average CSP rate is $9,080 per year. Average cost for the degree for international students is $200,000.

- Marks required:

  ○ ATAR or equivalent of 95.5 (or 93.5 for residents of Greater Western Sydney), or a GPA of 5.5

  ○ UMAT scores are not made public, as they vary with the performance of the applicants

- Contact details:

  ○ www.uws.edu.au/medicine/som

  ○ Phone: (02) 9852 4632

  ○ Fax: (02) 9852 4700

  ○ Email: medstudent@uws.edu.au

Monash University

- Monash University campuses are located in Clayton (18km from the CBD) and Gippsland (19km from the CBD) in Victoria, and in Malaysia. Cost of living is very low in Gippsland, moderate in Clayton and very high in Malaysia (rated as 11/5!).

- They offer 258 places, of which there are 190 Commonwealth Supported Places, 62 Bonded Places, and 6 Medical Rural Bonded Places.

- The medical degree is 5 years' duration.

- Rural schools include Mildura, Bendigo, Gippsland and East Gippsland.

- Their main focus is producing excellent doctors with an emphasis on research.

- Gippsland has 2,011 students, Clayton 23, 500, and the university itself ranks reasonably well academically. It is not part of the Australian or world ranking system.

- Comparisons with other Australian medical schools are not available.

- Average CSP rate is $9,080 per year. Average cost for the degree for international students is $246,000.

- Marks required:

  ○ ATAR or equivalent of 95 to be competitive (the minimum ATAR is 90)

- UMAT scores are not made public, as they vary with the performance of the applicants
- Contact details:
  - www.med.monash.edu.au
  - Phone: (03) 9905 4327
  - Fax: (03) 9905 9327
  - Email: medicineadmissions@med.monash.edu.au

University of Adelaide

- The University of Adelaide is located in North Terrace, Adelaide, which is 1km from the CBD. However, cost of accommodation is low.
- They offer 150 places, of which there are between 103 and 108 Commonwealth Supported Places, 35 to 40 Bonded Places (these numbers change each year) and 7 Medical Rural Bonded Places.
- The medical degree is 6 years' duration.
- Rural school is in the Spencer Gulf.
- Their main focus is producing excellent doctors with an emphasis on research.
- North Terrace has 18,650 students, and the university itself ranks well academically. In fact, it ranks 8th in Australia, and 201–225 in the world.
- Compared with other Australian medical schools, graduates rank teaching quality as average, generic skills as better than average, and overall satisfaction as average.
- Average CSP rate is $9,080 per year. Average cost for the degree for international students is $286,800.
- Marks required:
  - ATAR or equivalent of at least 90 (but average TER is over 99)
  - UMAT scores are not made public, as they vary with the performance of the applicants
- Contact details:
  - www.health.adelaide.edu.au
  - Phone: (08) 8303 4859
  - Fax: (08) 8303 3788
  - Email: admissions.health@adelaide.edu.au

Bond University

- Bond University is located in Robina in the Gold Coast, Queensland. This is 98km from the CBD and cost of accommodation is moderate.
- They offer 84 full-fee-paying places.
- The medical degree is 4 years and 8 months duration.
- Bond University does not have a rural clinical school.
- Their main focus is producing excellent doctors.
- Robina has 3,306 students, and the university itself ranks reasonably well academically. It is not part of the Australian or world ranking system.
- Comparisons with other Australian medical schools are not available.
- Average fee for all students (for the whole degree) is $298,918.
- Marks required:
  - ATAR or equivalent of 96, or a GPA of 6
  - UMAT total raw score of over 150
- Contact details:
  - www.bond.edu.au/hsm/medicine
  - Phone: 1800 074 074
  - Email: information@bond.edu.au

James Cook University

- James Cook University is located in Douglas, Townsville, which is 13km from the CBD. Cost of living is low.
- They offer 150 places, including 10–15 for graduate entry.
- The medical degree is 6 years' duration.
- Rural clinical schools include Darwin, Cairns and Mackay.
- Their main focus is producing excellent doctors who are able to contribute to rural practice.
- JCU has 7,631 students, and the university itself ranks reasonably well academically. It is not part of the Australian or world ranking system.
- Compared with other Australian medical schools, JCU graduates rank teaching quality as better than average, generic skills as average and overall satisfaction as better than average.

- Average CSP rate is $9,080 per year. Average cost for the degree for international students is $216,000.

- Marks required:
    - ATAR marks (or equivalent) are not released by the university, but the GPA required is 5.75.
    - The UMAT is not used for selection by James Cook University.

- Contact details:
    - www-public.jcu.edu.au/courses/course_info/index.htm?user Text=72010-&mainContent=detail and www.jcu.edu.au/fmhms/forms/index.htm
    - Phone: (07) 4781 6232

- Email: medicine@jcu.edu.au

University of Tasmania

- The University of Tasmania is located in Sandy Bay, Tasmania, which is 5km from the CBD. Cost of living is low.

- They offer 120 places, 75 of which are Commonwealth Supported Places, 25 are Bonded Places, and 20 are international places.

- The medical degree is 5 years' duration.

- Rural schools are located in Launceston and Burnie.

- Their main focus is producing excellent doctors.

- The UTAS campus has 10,196 students, and the university itself ranks reasonably well academically. In fact, it is ranked 15th in Australia, and 301–350 in the world

- Comparisons with other Australian medical schools are not available.

- Average CSP rate is $9,080 per year. Average cost for the degree for international students is $205,000.

- Marks required:
    - TER or equivalent of 90
    - UMAT total raw score of over 150

- Contact details:
    - www.healthsci.utas.edu.au
    - Phone: 1300 363 864

○ Fax: 03 6226 2087

○ Email: Course.Info@utas.edu.au

University of Otago

- Admission into medicine at the University of Otago is different to most Australian medical schools. To gain entry into medicine, you must complete the Health Sciences First Year (HSFY), from where you apply for admission to the 'Second Year Professional Programmes', which include medicine (see below for entry requirements for each step).

- You must be an Australian (or New Zealand) citizen to study at the University of Otago.

- The University of Otago is located in Dunedin, Otago, which is the second largest city on the South Island of New Zealand. Cost of living is moderate.

- Otago offers 210 spots per year, with 150 available for entry from the HSFY program, 40 via graduate entry, and 20 for Maori and Pacific Island students.

- The medical degree is 6 years' duration.

- Rural schools include Christchurch and Wellington.

- Their main focus is producing excellent doctors with an emphasis on research.

- The University of Otago has 22,000 students, and the university itself ranks well academically. It ranked within the top 201–225 in the world in 2011.

- Comparisons with Australian medical schools are not available.

- Average cost is $12,766 per year. Note that Australian students may not have access to the same payment deferral schemes as New Zealand students.

- <u>Marks required</u>:

    1. Entry onto the HSFY Program:

        - Applicants must achieve a high school leavers mark of 80 to be competitive

        - To apply for admission, students must register with the University of Otago. For registration materials and information, see www.otago.ac.nz/study/enrolling.html

    2. Entry onto the Medical Degree:

- Applicants must gain a B grade (70 percent) or better in all seven compulsory HSFY subjects and sit the UMAT
- Selection is determined using a combination of a student's Grade Point Average in the HSFY course (two-thirds) and their UMAT score (one-third)
- Contact details:
  - www.otago.ac.nz/courses/qualifications/mbchb.html#int
  - http://healthsci.otago.ac.nz/admissio0ns/pp_guidelines.html
  - Phone: (+64 3) 479 7000 (or 0800 80 80 98 within NZ)
  - Fax: (+64 3) 479 5058
  - Email: health-sciences@otago.ac.nz

Graduate Medical Schools

University of Sydney

- The University of Sydney is located in Camperdown, Sydney, which is 4km from Sydney CBD, or a 5 minute bus from Central Station. Cost of living is high.
- They offer 228 places, of which there are 163 Commonwealth Supported Places, 57 Bonded Places and 8 Medical Rural Bonded Places.
- The medical degree is 4 years' duration.
- Rural schools include Dubbo, Orange and Bathurst.
- Their main focus is producing excellent doctors with an emphasis on research,
- Camperdown campus has 34,468 students and the university itself ranks very well academically, ranking 3rd in Australia, and 58th in the world. In fact, it is the oldest and possibly the most prestigious medical school in Australia.
- Compared with other Australian medical schools, graduates rank Sydney University as average for teaching quality, generic skills and overall satisfaction.
- Average CSP rate is $9,080 per year. Average cost for the degree for international students is $237,120.

- NOTE: Applicants apply directly to the University of Sydney, not via ACER (this is the only graduate medical school that does not have its application process in conjunction with ACER).

- <u>Marks required</u>:
  - GPA of 5.5
  - GAMSAT score of 67

- <u>Contact details</u>:
  - http://sydney.edu.au/medicine/future-students/medical-program/index.php
  - Phone: (02) 9351 3132
  - Fax: (02) 9351 3196
  - Email: medicine.info@sydney.edu.au

University of Notre Dame (Sydney)

- The University of Notre Dame (Sydney) is located in Darlinghurst, Sydney. This is 1km from the CBD, or a 5 minute bus from Central Station. Cost of living is very high.

- They offer 112 places, of which there are 43 Commonwealth Supported Places, 15 Bonded Places, 2 Medical Rural Bonded Places and 52 full-fee-paying places.

- The medical degree is 4 years' duration.

- Rural schools include Wagga Wagga and Lithgow in New South Wales, and Melbourne and Ballarat in Victoria.

- Their main focus is producing excellent doctors in the context of Catholic values.

- The Darlinghurst campus has 1,000 students, and the university itself ranks well academically. It is not part of the Australian or world ranking system.

- Compared with other Australian medical schools, UNDA (Sydney) graduates rate teaching quality as average, and generic skills and overall satisfaction as average

- Average CSP rate is $9,080 per year. There are no spots for international students, and full-fee-paying students will pay around $100,000 for their degree.

- Marks required:
  - GPA of 5.0
  - GAMSAT score of 50
- Contact details:
  - www.nd.edu.au/sydney/schools/medicine/ugcourse.shtml
  - Phone: (02) 8204 4404
  - Email: sydney@nd.edu.au

University of Wollongong

- The University of Wollongong is located in Keiraville, Wollongong. This is 3km from the CBD, and cost of living is low.
- They offer 84 places, of which there are 51 Commonwealth Supported Places, 18 Bonded Places, 3 Medical Rural Bonded Places and 12 international places
- The medical degree is 4 years' duration.
- Rural schools include Shoalhaven North and South, the Southern Highlands, Murrumbidgee, Mudgee, Broken Hill and North Coast.
- Their main focus is producing excellent doctors, especially to work in rural and remote communities.
- The UOW has 16,716 students, and the university itself ranks well academically. In fact, it ranks 10th in Australia, and 251–275 in the world.
- Comparisons with other Australian medical schools are not available.
- Average CSP rate is $9,080 per year. Average cost for the degree for international students is $173,200.
- Marks required:
  - GPA of 5.0
  - GAMSAT scores of 50 in each section
- Contact details:
  - www.uow.edu.au/gsm/index.html
  - Phone: 1300 367 869
  - Email: uniadvice@uow.edu.au

University of Melbourne

- The University of Melbourne is located in Parkville, Melbourne, which is 3km from the CBD. Cost of living is very high.

- They offer 335 places, of which there are 183 Commonwealth Supported Places, 64 Bonded Places, 8 Medical Rural Bonded Places and 80 full-fee paying places.

- The medical degree is 4 years' duration.

- Rural schools include Shepparton, Ballarat, Bendigo and Wangaratta.

- Their main focus is producing excellent doctors, with an emphasis on research.

- Parkville campus has 30,000 students, and the university itself ranks very well academically. In fact, it is ranked as the top university in Australia and 37th in the world.

- Comparisons with other Australian medical schools are not available.

- Average CSP rate is $9,080 per year. Average cost for the degree for full-fee-paying students is $228,687.

- Marks required:
  - GPA of 5.0
  - GAMSAT scores of 50 in each section

- Contact details:
  - www.mdhs.unimelb.edu.au
  - Phone: (03) 8344 5890
  - Fax: (03) 9347 7084
  - Email: mdhs-sc@unimelb.edu.au

Monash University

- Monash University is located in Clayton, Melbourne. This is 18km from the CBD, with cost of living being moderate.

- They offer 85 places, of which there are 46 Commonwealth Supported Places, 16 Bonded Places, 3 Medical Rural Bonded Places, and 20 international places

- The medical degree is 4 years' duration.

- Rural schools include Mildura, Bendigo, Warragul, Sale, Traralgon and Bairnsdale.

- Their main focus is producing excellent doctors.

- Clayton has 23,500 students and the university itself ranks reasonably well academically. In fact, it is ranked 5th in Australia and 117th in the world.

- Comparisons with other Australian medical schools are not available.

- Average CSP rate is $9,080 per year. Average cost for the degree for international students is $246,000.

- Marks required:

    o GPA of 5.0

    o GAMSAT scores of 50 in each section

- Contact details:

    o www.med.monash.edu.au/medical/gippsland

    o Phone: (03) 5122 6445

    o Fax: (03) 5122 6841

    o Email: gippslandmed@monash.edu

Deakin University

- Deakin University is located in Waurn Ponds, Geelong, which is 10km from the CBD. Cost of living is low.

- They offer 146 places, of which there are 94 Commonwealth Supported Places, 32 Bonded Places, 4 Medical Rural Bonded Places, and 16 international places.

- The medical degree is 4 years' duration.

- Rural schools include Warrnambool, Box Hill and Ballarat.

- Their main focus is producing excellent doctors to practice in rural areas.

- Deakin has 4,368 students and the university itself ranks well academically. In fact, it is ranked 18th in Australia and 351–400 in the world.

- Comparisons with other Australian medical schools are not available.

- Average CSP rate is $9,080 per year. Average cost for the degree for international students is $209,160.

- Marks required:

- ○ GPA of 5.0
- ○ GAMSAT score of 50, with a minimum of 50 in each section
- Contact details:
  - ○ www.deakin.edu.au/hmnbs/medicine/admission.php
  - ○ Phone: (03) 9251 7777
  - ○ Fax: (03) 9251 7450
  - ○ Email: hmnbs-support@deakin.edu.au

Flinders University

- Flinders University is located in Bedford Park, Adelaide, which is 10km from the CBD. Cost of living is low.
- They offer 131 places, of which there are 56 Commonwealth Supported Places, 27 Bonded Places, 4 Medical Rural Bonded Places and 20 international places. There are also 24 Bonded Places in Darwin.
- The medical degree is 4 years' duration.
- Rural schools include the Barossa Valley, the Riverland and Mount Gambier.
- Their main focus is producing excellent doctors to practice in rural areas.
- Flinders University has 12,886 students and the university itself ranks reasonably well academically. In fact, it ranks 19th in Australia and 351–400 in the world.
- Compared with other Australian medical schools, graduates rank Flinders as average for teaching quality and generic skills, but better than average for overall satisfaction.
- Average CSP rate is $9,080 per year. Average cost of the degree for international students is $180,000.
- Marks required:
  - ○ There is no minimum GPA
  - ○ GAMSAT minimum scores range from 57 to 61
- Contact details:
  - ○ www.flinders.edu.au/medicine/sites/medical-course/medicine_home. cfm
  - ○ Phone: (08) 8201 2538
  - ○ Fax: (08) 8201 3905
  - ○ Email: medadmissions@flinders.edu.au

University of Queensland

- The University of Queensland is located in Herston (3km from the CBD) and St Lucia (4km from the CBD), Brisbane (and cost of living in both is moderate). A UQ medical school is also found in Ipswitch (40km from the CBD), which has a very low cost of living.

- They offer 429 places, of which there are 210 Commonwealth Supported Places, 75 Bonded Places, 14 Medical Rural Bonded Places and 130 international places

- The medical degree is 4 years' duration.

- Rural schools include Bundaberg, Hervey Bay, Rockhampton and Toowoomba.

- Their main focus is producing excellent doctors.

- The St Lucia campus has 33,477 students, and Ipswitch 1,918. The university itself ranks well academically, in fact is ranked 4th in Australia and 74th in the world.

- Compared with other Australian medical schools, graduates rank UQ as average for generic skills, and worse than average for teaching quality and overall satisfaction.

- Average CSP rate is $9,080 per year. Average cost for the degree for international students is $199,600.

- Marks required:
  - GPA of 5.0
  - GAMSAT scores of 50 in each section

- Contact details:
  - www.som.uq.edu.au
  - Phone: (07) 3365 5278
  - Fax: (07) 3365 5433
  - Email: admissions@som.uq.edu.au

Griffith University

- Griffith University is located in Southport, on the Gold Coast. This is 70km from the CBD. Cost of living is moderate.

- They offer 125 places, of which there are 92 Commonwealth Supported Places, 30 Bonded Places and 3 Medical Rural Bonded Places.

- The medical degree is 4 years' duration.

- Rural schools include Warwick, Kingaroy, Stanthorpe, Dalby, Oakey, Millmerran, Inglewood, Chinchilla, Gatton and Goondiwindi.

- Their main focus is producing excellent doctors.

- Southport has 12,768 students and the university itself ranks reasonably well academically. In fact, it ranks 20th in Australia and 351–400 in the world.

- Comparisons with other Australian medical schools are not available.

- Average CSP rate is $9,080 per year.

- Marks required:

  ○ GPA of 5.0

  ○ GAMSAT score of 50 in each section (scores are usually in the mid 60s)

- Contact details:

  ○ www.griffith.edu.au/health/school-medicine

  ○ Phone: (07) 5678 0704

  ○ Fax: (07) 5678 0303

  ○ Email: medicine@griffith.edu.au

University of Western Australia

- The University of Western Australia is located in Crawley, Perth. This is 5km from the CBD, and cost of living is moderate.

- They offer 60 places, of which there are 38 Commonwealth Supported Places, 15 Bonded Places and 7 Medical Rural Bonded Places.

- The medical degree is 4 years' duration.

- Rural schools are run in collaboration with the University of Notre Dame (Fremantle), and include Albany, Broome, Bunbury, Busselton, Carnarvon, Derby, Esperance, Geraldton, Kalgoorlie, Karratha, Kununurra, Narrogin and Port Hedland.

- Their main focus is producing excellent doctors.

- UWA has 20,000 students and the university itself ranks well academically. In fact, it is ranked 7th in Australia and 189th in the world.

- Comparisons with other Australian medical schools are not available.

- Average CSP rate is $9,080 per year.

- Marks required:
  - ○ GPA of 5.5
  - ○ GAMSAT scores of 50 in each section
- Contact details:
  - ○ www.meddent.uwa.edu.au/admissions
  - ○ Phone: (08) 6488 8500
  - ○ Email: meddentadmissions@uwa.edu.au

University of Notre Dame (Fremantle)

- The University of Notre Dame (Fremantle) is located in Fremantle, Perth. This is 19km from the CBD, and cost of living is moderate.
- They offer 100 places, of which there are 72 Commonwealth Supported Places, 25 Bonded Places and 3 Medical Rural Bonded Places.
- The medical degree is 4 years' duration.
- Rural schools are run in collaboration with the University of Western Australia, and include Narrogin, Bunbury, Geraldton, Kalgoorlie, Broome, Port Hedland, Karratha, Albany, Esperance and Derby.
- Their main focus is producing excellent doctors in the context of Catholic values.
- The Fremantle campus has 5,138 students, and the university itself ranks well academically. It is not part of the Australian or world ranking system.
- Compared with other Australian medical schools, UNDA (Fremantle) graduates rate teaching quality as average, and generic skills and overall satisfaction as average.
- Average CSP rate is $9,080 per year. There are no spots for international students, and full-fee-paying students will pay around $100,000 for their degree.
- Marks required:
  - ○ GPA of 5.0
  - ○ GAMSAT scores of 50 in each section
- Contact details:
  - ○ www.nd.edu.au/fremantle/courses/undergraduate/medicine/mbbs. shtml
  - ○ Phone: (08) 9433 0540
  - ○ Email: admissions@nd.edu.au

Australian National University

- The Australian National University is located in Acton, Canberra, which is 1km from the CBD. Cost of living is moderate.

- They offer 110 places, of which there are 64 Commonwealth Supported Places, 23 Bonded Places, 3 Medical Rural Bonded Places and 20 international places.

- The medical degree is 4 years' duration.

- Rural schools include Goulburn, Young, Eurobodalla, Bega and Cooma.

- Their main focus is producing excellent doctors, especially for practice in rural areas.

- ANU has 16,630 students and the university itself ranks well academically. In fact, it ranks second in Australia and 38th in the world.

- Compared with other Australian medical schools, graduating students rank teaching quality and generic skills as average, and overall satisfaction better than average.

- Average CSP rate is $9,080 per year. Average cost for the degree for international students is $216,192.

- Marks required:
  - GPA of 5.5
  - GAMSAT score of 55

- Contact details:
  - http://medicalschool.anu.edu.au
  - Phone: (02) 6125 1304
  - Fax: (02) 6125 8877
  - Email: medadmissions@anu.edu.au

University of Otago

- Admission into medicine at the University of Otago is different compared to most. Australian medical schools:
  - To gain entry into graduate medicine (under the spots reserved for 'Competitive Graduates', you must have obtained a university degree in New Zealand within three years).

○ Alternatively, you can gain entry under the 'Other' category, which requires a previous degree, plus health-related professional experience (including academic) of a minimum of two years.

- You must be an Australian (or New Zealand) citizen to study at the University of Otago.

- The University of Otago is located in Dunedin in Otago, which is the second largest city on the South Island of New Zealand. Cost of living is moderate.

- Otago offers 210 spots per year, with 150 available for entry from the HSFY program, 40 for graduate entry and 20 for Maori and Pacific Island students.

- The medical degree is 6 years' duration, with graduates entering at second year.

- Rural schools include Christchurch and Wellington.

- Their main focus is producing excellent doctors with an emphasis on research.

- The University of Otago has 22,000 students and the university itself ranks well academically. It ranked within the top 201–225 in the world in 2011.

- Comparisons with Australian medical schools are not available.

- Average cost is $12,766 per year. Note that Australian students may not have access to the same payment deferral schemes as New Zealand students.

- Marks required:

  ○ Applicants offered a place under the 'Competitive Graduates' or 'Other' categories may be required to satisfy academic bridging requirements or pass prerequisite papers at a standard to be determined by the Medical Admissions Committee, before being admitted to second year classes.

  ○ Contact the university for more information

- Contact details:

  ○ www.otago.ac.nz/courses/qualifications/mbchb.html#int

  ○ http://healthsci.otago.ac.nz/admissions/pp_guidelines.html

  ○ Phone: (+64 3) 479 7000 (or 0800 80 80 98 within NZ)

  ○ Fax: (+64 3) 479 5058

  ○ Email: health-sciences@otago.ac.nz

A | Practice UMAT Questions

Section 1 – Logical Reasoning and Problem Solving

Question 1

Relationships between two organisms include:

- <u>Commensalism</u> – one organism benefits, and the other neither benefits nor is harmed
- <u>Mutualism</u> – both organisms benefit from the interaction
- <u>Parasitism</u> – one organism benefits at the expense of the other
- <u>Amensalism</u> – one organism is harmed, and the other neither benefits nor is harmed

1) <u>The best term to describe the relationship between a spider that builds its web in a tree and the tree is</u>:

   A. Commensalism

   B. Mutualism

   C. Parasitism

   D. Amensalism

Questions 2–3

The following questions are based on the following paragraph:

'Sustained ventricular tachycardia (VT) is a heart rhythm where the ventricles (the two larger pumping chambers of the heart) beat at a rate of greater than 100 beats per minute, which either lasts for over 30 seconds or causes haemodynamic compromise (any of low blood pressure, chest pain, or loss of consciousness), with specific changes seen on electrocardiogram (ECG). It is due to an extra connection between the conducting system of the atria and ventricles, causing normal conduction of the heart to be altered. If the patient is haemodynamically compromised, they require

defibrillation (shocks with electricity). If the patient is haemodynamically stable (which means their circulation is fine and not compromised) they are given drugs, have the extra-conducting connection removed, or have an implantable defibrillator inserted, which gives shocks if needed.'

2) <u>Tony is brought into the emergency department by ambulance after being found collapsed in a shopping mall, and the ambulance officers performed an ECG and found he had VT. He has not woken up since his collapse. What treatment is needed?</u>

    A. Defibrillation

    B. Drugs

    C. Removal of the extra-conducting pathway

    D. Insertion of an implantable defibrillator

3) <u>Janet has recently undergone removal of an extra-conducting pathway in her heart. Her heart rate would previously reach 150 beats per minute, lasting for hours at a time, but is now 70 most of the time. What was her previous diagnosis?</u>

    A. Ventricular tachycardia

    B. Ventricular tachycardia requiring defibrillation

    C. Ventricular tachycardia requiring drug treatment

    D. Not enough information is given

Questions 4–6

The following questions refer to the two graphs below:

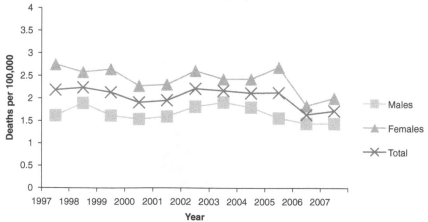

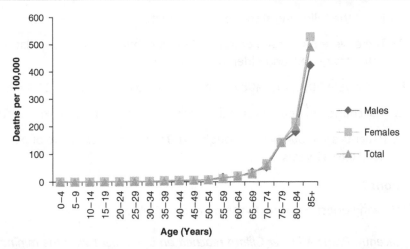

Deaths due to pulmonary embolism in Australia, from 1997 to 2007. Data is taken from the 'AIHW General Record of Incidence of Mortality Books'. Canberra: Australian Institute of Health and Welfare, 2010.

4) The population of the city of Sydney was estimated to be 4.25 million in 2005; 50 percent male, 50 percent female. From the graph, estimate how many deaths in females living in Sydney in 2005 were due to pulmonary embolism?

   A. 60

   B. 120

   C. 2.7

   D. 6.3

5) The graphs suggest that:

   A. Mortality from pulmonary embolism is increasing over time

   B. Deaths from pulmonary embolism were greater in males in 1999 than females in 2007

   C. Risk of death from a pulmonary embolism decreases with age

   D. Males and females have a similar trend over time in deaths from pulmonary embolism

6) <u>Which of the following statements is correct?</u>

    A. There were more total deaths in females than the total population in patients aged 85 and older in 1997 to 2007

    B. In the year 2000, the ratio of male to female deaths was 3 : 2.25

    C. The change in death rate with age could be described as exponential

    D. Patients aged 80–84 have roughly 200 times the death rate of patients aged 0 to 49 years

Questions 7–8

The following questions refer to the paragraph below:

'Recently, Prime Minister Gillard reached an agreement with the mining industry regarding an alternative to the proposed super-profits tax. The agreement involved the creation of the Mineral Resource Rent Tax, which applies to companies mining coal and iron ore, and only those making a $50 million profit. This comes after a heated debate about whether the resources taken from Australian land should be distributed amongst Australians, or should end up in the pockets of mining companies. However, these mining companies have always been subject to taxes, so have been paying their way for years. The opposition is worried that Gillard's moves may be lethal to the mining industry.'

7) <u>From the information given, which company will suffer the LEAST loss of profits?</u>

    A. A company mining coal, making $50 million per year

    B. A company mining nickel, making $100 million per year

    C. A company mining iron ore, making $100 million per year

    D. A company mining coal and iron ore, making $50 million per year

8) <u>The recent change in the mining tax is due to:</u>

    A. The government wanting a bigger share of profits

    B. A general feeling that Australia should profit, not just the mining companies

    C. Companies making less than $50 million were paying too much tax

    D. There is not much coal and iron ore, so it needs to be taxed more heavily

Questions 9–10

The following questions refer to the paragraph below:

'Technology and the internet have improved many aspects of life, including our health. We are able to use the internet to search for locations of local medical practitioners and read about people with similar health experiences to ours, and the available technologies (such as CT and MRI) have improved medical diagnosis dramatically. However, there is a dark side. People are using internet search engines to search for answers to their medical illnesses, and smartphone applications provide a similar service. This not only has health implications, but possibly legal ones too. Creators of smart-phone applications are likely to be fair game to be held liable in the case of misdiagnosis or injury, just as the creator of a new medication or medical device would be held liable.'

9) <u>What is the author's main argument in this paragraph?</u>

A. Technology and the internet have improved our health, as well as our understanding of how we and others experience illness

B. The internet is to blame for many misdiagnoses

C. Smartphone applications may risk the health of the patient, and the designers may then be sued

D. The internet, smartphone applications, CT and MRI all have positives and negatives

10) <u>What would NOT be one way the smartphone application designers could help prevent misdiagnosis and harm?</u>

A. For all symptoms, list one possible life-threatening cause and encourage people to seek a doctor if they are concerned

B. Program the application so when it is turned on, a warning says 'Users use this application at their own risk'

C. Be extremely accurate, taking into account the individual patients data such as heart rate and blood pressure

D. Have a doctor available 24 hours, that a user can call if concerned

Answers

1) A spider gains benefit from having its web in the tree, while the tree is unlikely to be affected. This makes A correct, and the others (B, C and D) incorrect.

2) The correct answer is A, as he was found collapsed and has not woken up, which means that the ventricular tachycardia has caused haemodynamic compromise (we are told that haemodynamic compromise includes loss of consciousness). This requires you to quickly work out that the words 'collapse' and 'has not woken up' mean loss of consciousness, and that we are told loss of consciousness → haemodynamic compromise → defibrillation. The other answers are for patients who are haemodynamically stable.

3) The correct answer is D. We are told that she has symptoms that may have indicated VT, but we are not given enough information to tell this for sure (for example, we are not told what the ECG showed). Thus, we know it *could* have been VT, but it could also have been something else so we cannot say for sure without further information, making A, B and C incorrect.

4) The correct answer is A. You can work this out as follows:

   a. The rate of deaths in females in Sydney due to pulmonary embolism in 2005 was around 2.7 per 100,000.

   b. In 2005, the population of Sydney was 4.25 million, and 50 percent were female, meaning there were 2.125 million females in Sydney in 2005. Since we are given the rate per 100,000, this is 2, 125,000 females.

   c. The death rate is 2.7 per 100,000 females, and there were 2,125,000 females, which means we need to multiply 2.7 by 21.15 (as 2,125,000 divided by 100,000 is 21.25), giving us 57.4.

   d. So, the number of females that died from a pulmonary embolism in 2005 in Sydney is around 57, which is closest to A, 60

5) The correct answer is D: A is incorrect as rates are decreasing, B is incorrect as deaths from pulmonary embolism were less in males in 1999 than females in 2007, and C is incorrect as risk of death from a pulmonary embolism increases with age.

6) The correct answer is C, as the shape of the curve in the second graph is exponential. A is incorrect, as although the second graph demonstrates that female death rates per 100,000 are higher than total death rates, this

is demonstrating rates per 100,000 and not total rates. Total rates would obviously include the female death rate plus the male death rate, which would be more than the total female rate. B is incorrect, as the correct ratio would be 6:9.

7) The correct answer is B, as a company making nickel is not subject to the tax, so its profits will remain unchanged. Any company mining coal (A), iron ore (C) or both (D) stand to suffer from the implementation of this tax. Be careful to notice the word *least* when you read the question. It often helps to circle, underline or highlight it, because it would be awful to forget or ignore it when re-reading the question after you have searched for the answer in the text.

8) The correct answer is B, which is seen in the sentence '*This comes after a heated debate about whether the resources taken from Australian land should be distributed amongst Australians, or should end up in the pockets of mining companies*'. The governments wish for profits is not discussed (A), and we are not told the reason for the $50 million threshold (C). While D may or may not be true, we are not told the reason for these commodities being taxed more heavily, and thus cannot choose D as the correct answer.

9) The correct answer is C. While the paragraph begins discussing the positives of technology and the internet (A), it goes on to focus on smart phones and the legal implications, making C correct. Searching for medical illnesses is mentioned (B), but isn't the main argument. Also, while it is mentioned that the various technologies have benefits, the negatives of CT and MRI are not discussed, making D incorrect.

10) The correct answer is B, as this warning may protect the company from legal action, but would not prevent misdiagnosis and harm, which is what the question is asking. The other answers are all true, and so are not the right answer (again, be careful with words like *not* and *least* in the question).

Section 2 – Understanding People

Questions 1–2

Your friend has been finding it increasingly hard to breathe for several hours now, and you take him to the hospital. They diagnose him with pneumonia, and send him home with antibiotics. However, once home, his symptoms worsen and he is admitted to hospital with all of the clinical hallmarks of an asthma attack.

1) <u>How does your friend most likely feel?</u>

    A. Well looked after by the hospital staff

    B. That the first doctor lied to him

    C. Unsure of his diagnosis

    D. Untrusting of the first doctor

2) <u>What is the best way to make your friend feel better?</u>

    A. Bring him whatever he feels like from the hospital cafeteria

    B. Tell him you understand he is concerned about his situation, and that you will remain with him in hospital, and talk with the doctors about the initial misdiagnosis

    C. Tell him you are worried about him, and that he should sue the first doctor

    D. Tell him you will go home and look after his things

Questions 3–5

A classmate has been having trouble at home, and so is struggling to keep up with schoolwork. She later asks you to help her cheat on the upcoming exam.

3) <u>How do you feel about her troubles?</u>

    A. Wish she hadn't burdened you with her problems

    B. Feel sorry for her and wish you could help

    C. Think she should work harder to keep up

    D. Think she should run away from home

4) <u>What should you do about helping her cheat with the exam?</u>

    A. Help her because she is having difficulties at home, and she will then help you cheat on exams in the future

    B. Tell your teacher she is trying to cheat

    C. Talk to her, and tell her you aren't comfortable with cheating, but that you are happy to help her study for the exam

    D. Tell her to cheat from someone else

5) <u>You decline to help her, so she cheats off someone else. She does very well, and decides to keep cheating. What should you do?</u>

    a. Encourage her to talk to the counsellor about her troubles at home, assure her that the teachers will be keen to help her with her studies

    b. Become resigned to the fact that she is going to cheat, so stop hassling her about it

    c. Start cheating as she does, as she is getting good marks

    d. Tell the teacher she cheated

Question 6

Your friend is trying out for the same spot on the rugby team as you, and is likely to be chosen over you, even though you have been training for months.

6) <u>How do you feel about this?</u>

    A. You hope your friend hurts himself

    B. You encourage your friend to try out for another spot 'as it would suit him better'

    C. You are happy for your friend, but are a little upset that you missed out on the spot

    D. You are ecstatic for him, and don't mind missing out on selection

Questions 7–9

Answer the questions on the following exchange:

    PATIENT: *'The other nurses are putting poisons in my food.'*

    NURSE: *'No they aren't, Mr Smith.'*

    PATIENT: *'Yes they are, I've seen them. And who knows what these tablets are for?'*

    NURSE: *'Mr Smith, you are being paranoid. Stop causing a fuss.'*

7) <u>How is the nurse handling Mr Smith's concerns:</u>

    A. Professionally

    B. Quickly and decisively

    C. Empathically

    D. Poorly

8) <u>What is NOT a possible reason that the nurse is responding as she is</u>:

A. She is busy

B. She is very concerned about Mr Smith's psychological and physical health

C. Mr Smith is well known to be paranoid and anxious, and has a background of similar complaints

D. She is well known to have very little empathy for her patients

9) <u>What is the best response to when the patient says '*The other nurses are putting poisons in my food. I've seen them. And who knows what these tablets are for?*'</u>:

A. As the nurse in the exchange responded

B. Tell him it's possible, and you will check this for him

C. Assure him that this is not the case (and demonstrate this if possible), ask Mr Smith why he thinks this, and explain what each of his tablets are for

D. Explain the other nurses aren't very good at their job, and that the doctors often prescribe unnecessary medications

Question 10

10) <u>Seventeen-year-old Steve is 50 cents short of money to buy lunch, so he sneaks into his 22-year-old brother's room and goes through his things until he finds his wallet, and takes 50 cents from a big pile of coins. His brother (Daniel) comes home and is very angry with Steve, even though Steve has offered to pay him back. What is the most likely reason Daniel is angry with Steve?</u>

A. Daniel needs that 50 cents immediately

B. Daniel is very protective of his money

C. Steve went through Daniel's things, and took the money without asking

D. Daniel likes his property kept in the way it is, and hates people (especially Steve) moving it around

Answers

1) The answer is D, as your friend is now fairly sure that his diagnosis is asthma (C) as it has *'all of the clinical hallmarks of an asthma attack'*, and so most likely has no trust in the first doctor he saw. As the first diagnosis was incorrect, he does not feel well looked after (A), but the first doctor probably didn't lie to him (B), but instead got the diagnosis wrong.

2) The answer is B, as you are being empathic, staying with him and addressing his main concern of his misdiagnosis. Bringing him food (A) or looking after his things at home (D) don't address his main (life-threatening) concerns, and telling him to sue the doctor is unlikely to deal directly with his worries.

3) The correct answer is B, as she is finding life at home difficult and it is affecting her schoolwork, two things which you wish she didn't have to deal with. Only psychopaths could ignore her unfortunate situation and wish she hadn't burdened them with her troubles (A). It would be inappropriate to think she should deal with her problems by working harder (C) as this doesn't deal with her issues at home, or by running away from home (D).

4) The answer is C, as you are being open and honest with her, you are not helping her cheat and you are willing to assist her with her studies. You should not help her cheat (A). Running to the teacher (B) betrays the trust she has in you and you may be able to talk her out of cheating before resorting to this step, so is incorrect. Telling her to cheat from someone else (D) does not deal with the issue, but merely absolves you of responsibility.

5) The answer is A, as you are encouraging her to deal with her problems, as well as helping with her studies. B is incorrect as you are merely allowing her to continue to cheat, and C is incorrect as now you both are cheating. D is incorrect for the reasons mentioned in the answer to Question 4.

6) The correct answer is C, as you wish good things for your friend, but you had worked hard for months and have missed out. It would be wrong to hope he is injured (A) or lie to him in order to get on the team yourself (B). Since you worked hard, you do mind that you missed out, making D incorrect.

7) The nurse is not addressing Mr Smith's concerns (and is being quite rude), so the answer is D. She is not being empathic, professional, or dealing with his concerns, so A, B and C are incorrect.

8) The nurse may be busy (A), (s)he may act like this all the time (C), or may have absolutely no empathy (D), so B is the correct answer. Also, (s)he obviously doesn't care too much about Mr Smith's physical or mental health, so B is correct.

9) The best response would be to address the patients concerns and reassure him, so C is correct. The nurse in the exchange does not give a good response, so A is incorrect. Agreeing with his paranoia is not recommended, making B incorrect. Blaming other staff is always wrong, so D is incorrect.

10) The correct answer is C. It is unlikely that Daniel needs the 50 cents immediately (as we are told he already has a big pile of coins), making A incorrect. Steve has offered to pay Daniel back, so B is also incorrect (as it isn't about the money). It is possible that D is correct, but it is more likely that Daniel is upset at his privacy and trust in Steve (to not take property or money from him without asking) have been violated, making C correct.

Section 3 – Non-verbal Reasoning

1)

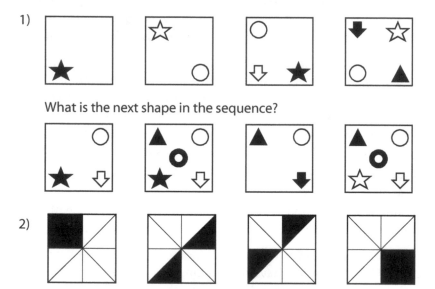

What is the next shape in the sequence?

2)

Arrange these shapes in order, and select the next shape in the sequence. The first shape has been done for you.

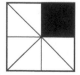 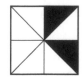

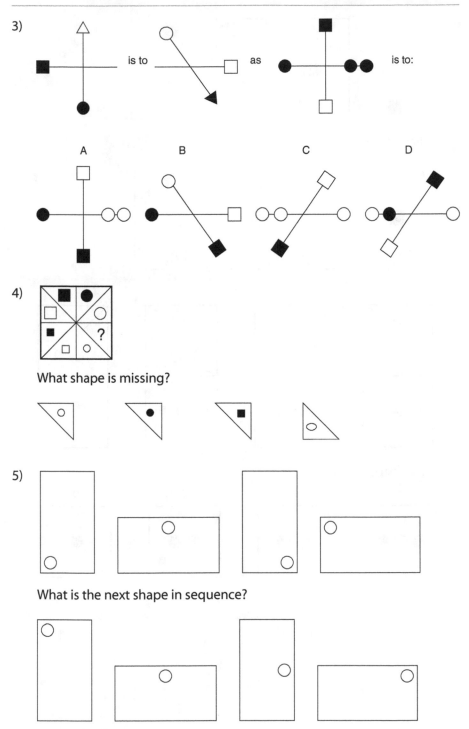

3)

A   B   C   D

4)

What shape is missing?

5)

What is the next shape in sequence?

6)

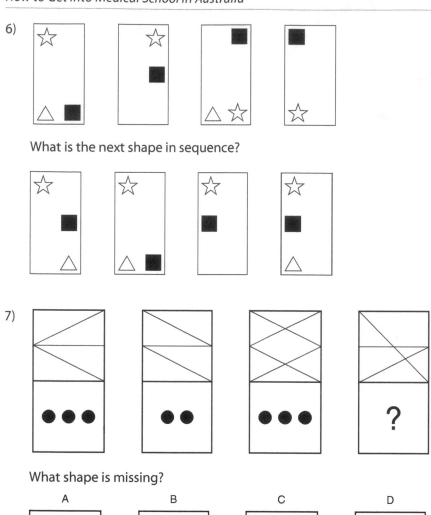

What is the next shape in sequence?

7)

What shape is missing?

A   B   C   D

8)

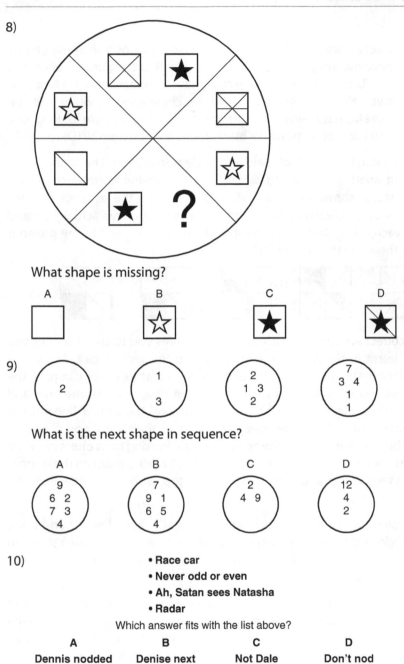

What shape is missing?

A   B   C   D

9)

What is the next shape in sequence?

A   B   C   D

10)
- **Race car**
- **Never odd or even**
- **Ah, Satan sees Natasha**
- **Radar**

Which answer fits with the list above?

A	**B**	**C**	**D**
Dennis nodded	**Denise next**	**Not Dale**	**Don't nod**

Answers

1) The correct answer is B. This is tricky, as it isn't the position of the objects which have meaning, but the number. Notice that the number of objects goes, 1, 2, 3, 4, so the next shape must have 5 objects, leaving B or D as the answer. However, see that while the circle remains white, the star and arrow alternate between white and black. Thus, you are looking for a shape that has 5 objects, with a black star and a white arrow (D).

2) This is a hard one, so look below for a demonstration. The triangles are moving apart (one moving clockwise, one moving counter-clockwise) each step, as shown by the arrows. The hard part is the last step, in which the shapes look like they haven't moved while they have actually crossed over each other, and are in the spot the other occupied in the previous step. Therefore the answer is D.

3) The correct answer is C. This question requires you to use the rules you have learnt in the first pair, and apply it to the second pair. As with all puzzles like this, note the number of different features – for example, the first pair has lines which rotate, shapes that swap ends of the lines and shapes that change colour. The first pair involves the vertical line moving diagonally, and the shapes swapping ends of their lines, and changing from black to white. Thus, the answer you are looking for is one with white circles (two on the left and one on the right), a black square on the bottom of the vertical line and a white one on the top, with the vertical line now diagonal (so C).

4) The correct answer is B. This is an easy one. On both the left and right, the circle and square are alternating black and white, and then shrink in the bottom square. This means you are looking for a black circle in a left-facing triangle, B.

5) The correct answer is C. Note that you have two features here; a moving rectangle and a moving circle. The rectangle is rotating clockwise each turn (not merely sitting up then down), while the circle is moving halfway each time, in the rotating rectangle. This is tough, as it makes you try and follow the circles progress in the rotating rectangle. Just keep practicing – they get easier the more you do!

6) The correct answer is D. You have 3 features, a triangle, square and star. The star is moving between each corner every time, while the square is moving one position (including into the middle) each time. The triangle is appearing and disappearing every time. So, you are looking for an answer with the star in the top left hand corner, square in the middle on the left and the triangle re-appeared on the bottom left.

7) This is a tricky one. The pattern is merely how many times the lines separately touch the right-hand side of the top box. This makes C the correct answer. B is incorrect as one of the circles is not filled in, unlike the preceding pattern.

8) The correct answer is A. You will notice the pattern is alternating triangles of stars and lines, with the stars merely changing colour and the lines adding one to the box each time. The empty triangle is a triangle with a square in it, which is part of the line pattern. Since the pattern is adding a line each time, this box must either have no lines (and be the start of the sequence) or have 4 lines – and since only the former option is available, A is the right answer.

9) The correct answer is B. The sequence is the total of the numbers, which is increasing by multiplying the previous number by 2. Since you start with 2, the next circle adds to 4, the next 8, the next 16, and the next shape should have numbers adding to 32 (which is answer B).

10) The correct answer is D. The list is a list of palindromes (words or phrases which read the same way backwards or forwards. The only answer fitting this criteria is answer D. This is a tough question!

B | Practice GAMSAT Questions

Section 1 – Reasoning in Humanities and Social Sciences

Questions 1–2

The following passage is taken from *The Waves*, by Virginia Wolf.

> *'Beneath us lie the lights of the herring fleet. The cliffs vanish. Rippling small, rippling grey, innumerable waves spread beneath us. I touch nothing. I see nothing. We may sink and settle on the waves. The sea will drum in my ears. The white petals will be darkened with sea water. They will float for a moment and then sink. Rolling me over the waves will shoulder me under. Everything falls in a tremendous shower, dissolving me.'*

1) <u>In talking about the 'waves', the character is describing</u>:

   A. The constant movement of the world

   B. The constant movement of the water

   C. The passage of time

   D. Freedom

2) <u>The overall tone of this passage gives the feeling of</u>:

   A. Freedom

   B. Despair

   C. Questioning the meaning of life

   D. Being blind

Questions 3–7

The following passages are taken from Leo Tolstoy's *Anna Karenina*.

> *'In that brief glance Vronsky had time to notice the restrained animation that played over her face and fluttered between her shining eyes and the*

barely noticeable smile that curved her red lips. It was as if a surplus of something so overflowed her being that it expressed itself beyond her will, now in the brightness of her glance, now in her smile.'

3) <u>The best summary of this passage would be</u>:

    A. Eyes being the window to the soul

    B. Confusion felt by Vronsky

    C. The heroine inwardly laughing at Vronsky

    D. A description of love at first sight

4) <u>The language used by Tolstoy can be described as</u>:

    A. Emotive

    B. Visually evocative

    C. Metaphorical

    D. Sarcastic

5) <u>Why did the author choose to use the phrase *'restrained'*, when discussing the characters animation?</u>

    A. It describes the restraint a woman of that time was expected to display in courtship

    B. The character did not feel any emotion towards Vronsky

    C. As juxtaposition against the extreme visual descriptions which follow

    D. To demonstrate that Vronsky was a good judge of character

"'No, you're going in vain," she mentally addressed a company in a coach-and-four who were evidently going out of town for some merriment. "And the dog you're taking with you won't help you. You won't get away from yourselves."'

6) <u>In this monologue, the character is</u>:

    A. Wishing she could warn the strangers about their predicament

    B. Assuming everyone feels like she does

    C. Being smug that she is aware of the right way to go about life

    D. Demonstrating that dogs are poor distractions from life

7) The phrase '*a company in a coach-and-four*' likely means:

   A. Some people in a carriage pulled by four horses

   B. A group of business-people in a highly regarded corporation

   C. Her friends who are leaving her

   D. A group of business colleagues in a bus with four wheels

Questions 8–10

The following passage is from *Moby Dick*, by Herman Melville:

'Towards thee I roll, thou all-destroying but unconquering whale; to the last I grapple with thee; from hell's heart I stab at thee; for hate's sake I spit my last breath at thee. Sink all coffins and all hearses to one common pool and since neither can be mine, let me then tow to pieces, while still chasing thee, though tied to thee, thou damned whale! Thus, I give up the spear!'

8) This monologue is likely delivered at which point?

   A. As the character is about to make his last attempt to catch the whale

   B. After the character retires from chasing the whale

   C. As the characters last words before death

   D. As the character is making macho threats in front of others

9) The wording chosen by Melville makes the phrasing seem:

   A. Defiant

   B. Regretful

   C. Conclusive

   D. Compromising

10) The phrase '*Thus, I give up the spear*' is NOT likely to mean:

   A. The character has stopped his chase

   B. The character is about to die

   C. The character is giving up the direction of his life

   D. The character has finally decided to not literally fight the devil

Answers

1) The character uses the motif of waves to describe the passage of time, which she feels is irresistible (*'rolling me over the waves will shoulder me under'*), and so the answer is C. This can also be seen when she discusses her *'dissolving'* in the water, suggestive of being dissolved in the passage of time. A is incorrect as there is no discussion of movement of the world, B is incorrect as the character is using the term *'waves'* as a symbol (also indicated by the phrasing of the question), and D is incorrect, as although tempting, having waves 'shoulder me under' sounds more repressive than freeing.

2) The passage overall gives the feeling of depression or despair, B. This is observed by the numerous references to sinking, being shouldered under the water, being dissolved and to darkness. There is nothing to suggest freedom (A) or questioning the meaning of life, and *'I touch nothing, I see nothing'* suggests more nothingness than being blind (D).

3) This passage is a classic description of love at first sight (D). While there is reference to eyes (A), and her animation and smile (which hints at C), these answers are not correct when the whole paragraph is read together. There is no hint at confusion by Vronsky (B).

4) The language used by Tolstoy is incredibly visually evocative (B), with words like *'brief glance'*, *'shining eyes'*, *'barely noticeable smile'*, *'curved her red lips'*. While emotions are obviously being felt by both characters, this is secondary to the images seen by the reader upon reading this passage (A). The passage is not a metaphor (C), nor is it sarcastic (D).

5) The use of the word *'restrained'* demonstrates the restraint that a woman of that time was expected to display (A). This can be inferred from the language, the culture in which the book was set, as well as the fact that B is obviously not true, C would counteract the authors aim of creating a very visual passage and there is nothing to suggest that Vronsky was a good judge of character (D).

6) The character appears to be 'projecting', or assuming that others are feeling as she does (B). A is incorrect, as from the passage we are given, there is no real predicament to warn others about. She doesn't seem smug (C), nor does she seem to be talking about dogs (D) (NB: the dog is used to mean any distraction people seek).

7) This answer requires you to know (or deduce from the era of the book) that a 'coach and four' is a carriage pulled by four horses (A), so B, C and D are incorrect.

8) This monologue is delivered as the characters last words (C). This can be seen with the phrases *'all-destroying'*, *'to the last'*, *'my last breath'*, *'coffins'*, *'hearses'* and *'I give up the spear'*. A and B are incorrect, as the character makes it clear he has not and will not give up trying to catch the whale (*'Towards thee I roll'*, *'while still chasing thee'*). No others are mentioned, and the monologue appears delivered at the whale itself, making D incorrect.

9) The words used, such as *'to the last'*, *'I grapple'*, *'while still chasing thee'* makes the monologue seem defiant (A), and definitely not compromising (D). There is no hint of regret (B), and as mentioned in the answer to Question 8 there is no talk of resolution or conclusion (C).

10) The phrase *'Thus, I give up the spear'* can mean that the character is giving up the chase and direction of his life against his wishes (A and C), and he is about to die (B). While hell is mentioned, there is no mention of literally fighting the devil, so D is incorrect. Many questions will have a 'NOT' in the question, which is bolded and capitalised, but is still easy to miss – read each question carefully!

Section 2 – Written Communication

You have 10 minutes reading time, and 60 minutes to write two essays. Choose one quote from Section 2A and one from Section 2B, and develop a piece of writing in response.

Section 2A

'The pursuit of truth and beauty is a sphere of activity in which we are permitted to remain children all our lives.'

—Albert Einstein

'Beauty is all very well at first sight; but who ever looks at it when it has been in the house three days?'

—George Bernard Shaw

'When I admire the wonders of a sunset or the beauty of the moon, my soul expands in the worship of the creator.'

—Mahatma Gandhi

'Everything has beauty, but not everyone sees it.'

—Confucius

'As we grow old, the beauty steals inward.'

—Ralph Waldo Emerson

Section 2B

'A day without an argument is like an egg without salt.'

—Angela Carter

'Argument is meant to reveal the truth, not to create it.'

—Edward de Bono

'Behind every argument is someone's ignorance.'

—Robert Benchley

'In argument, truth always prevails finally; in politics, falsehood always.'

—Walter Savage Landor

'No matter what side of the argument you are on, you always find people on your side that you wish were on the other.'

—Thomas Berger

Answers

The markers are looking for the quality of the ideas expressed, the organisation of the essay, and how it is said (that is, phrasing and grammar). Consider using more than one quote for each essay, especially if the quotes give opposing views. Remember that you are not obliged to agree with the quote – just choose the quote you feel (positively or negatively) most strongly about.

Section 3 – Reasoning in Biological and Physical Sciences

Question 1

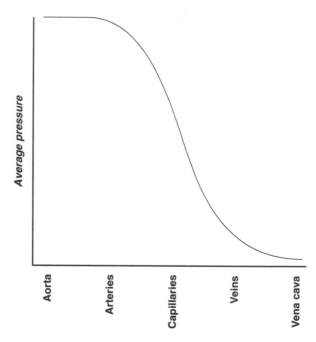

Flow pressures in the systemic human vasculature

1) <u>In the human body, where is the pressure drop the greatest?</u>

   A. Between the aorta and the capillaries

   B. Between the capillaries and veins

   C. Between the aorta and the arteries

   D. Between the veins and arteries

Questions 2–3

The torque (T) around an axis of rotation is the product of the perpendicular distance of the axis from the line of effect of the force (D), and the component of the force in the plane perpendicular to the axis (F). Torque is measured in Newton metres (Nm), distance in metres (m) and force in Newtons (N).

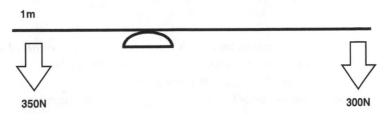

2) Force required to move a spanner around a screw is 5N, with the handle 20cm from the screw. What is the torque produced?

A. 0.1Nm

B. 1Nm

C. 5Nm

D. 10Nm

3) In the diagram of the see-saw above, a 350N force is 1m to the left of the fulcrum. How far is the 300N force on the right of the fulcrum to keep the see-saw balanced?

A. 10.66m

B. 1.35m

C. 1.17m

D. 0.82m

Questions 4–5

Table of cardioactive drugs

Drug	Receptor types involved in action	Effect on cardiac contractility	Effect on heart rate	Effect on blood pressure	Effect on constriction of the peripheral arteries and veins	Dose
Dopamine	DA_1, β_1, β_2, α	↑↑	↑	↑	↑	0.5–20µg/kg/min
Adrenaline	β_1, β_2, α	↑↑	↑	↑↑	↑	1–10µg/min
Noradrenaline	Mostly α, some β_1	-	-	↑↑	↑↑	0.5–1.5µg/kg/min
Dobutamine	Mostly β_1, some β_2, α	↑	↑	-	↓	2.5–20µg/kg/min

DA_1 = dopamine receptor 1, β_1 = beta receptor 1, β_2 = beta receptor 2, α = alpha receptor

Septic shock

>   'In septic shock, bacteria enter the bloodstream and release chemicals which cause the peripheral (not the vessels of the lungs, heart or brain) arteries and veins to dilatate. This reduces the blood pressure of the body, and can lead to death. Contraction of the cardiac muscle (heart) is unaffected.'

4) Which of the drugs from the table above would be most useful for a patient in septic shock?

A. Dopamine

B. Adrenaline

C. Noradrenaline

D. Dobutamine

5) A 60-year-old male (Giles Laurence) has had a cough and fever for 5 days, and is feeling progressively more tired. He presents to the hospital in septic shock. His blood pressure is 90/40, heart rate 120, respiratory rate 32 and he weighs 75kg. He lives in south Sydney with his wife and three children. He works 5 days a week as a banking executive, in a 60 storey office building in the centre of the city. What is the correct range of the appropriate drug to give Giles?

A. 37.5–112.5mg/kg

B. 37.5–1,500 µg/kg/min

C. 75–750µg/min

D. 37.5–112.5 µg/kg/min

Question 6

$$PV = nRT$$

The ideal gas law, where P = pressure (in kPa), V = volume (in cm^3), n = number of moles, R = 8.314, and T is temperature (in Kelvin)

6) 150g of CO_2 gas is placed into a 5L evacuated container at 100°C. How much O_2 gas would I have to add to a 3L evacuated container at the same temperature to achieve the same pressure? The atomic weight of carbon is 12, and the atomic weight of O_2 is 16.

A. 65.4g

B. 654.2g

C. 373g

D. 2.046g

Questions 7–8

7) <u>Which of these do NOT have an enantiomer?</u>

A.

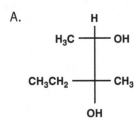

B.

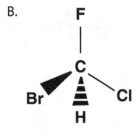

C.

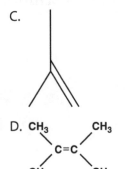

D.

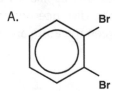

8) <u>Benzene plus 2Br produces which of the following reactions?</u>

A.

B.

Br + HBr

C.

Br$_2$

D. In benzene + 2Br, no reaction occurs

Questions 9–10

9) <u>Which of these equations are correctly balanced?</u>

A. $Ca + 2GdF_3 \rightarrow 2Gd + CaF_2$

B. $3C_2H_3OCl + 2O_2 \rightarrow 2CO + 2H_2O + HCl$

C. $P_4O_{10} + 6H_2O \rightarrow 4H_3PO_4$

D. $C_2H_5NSCl + 5O_2 \rightarrow 2CO_2 + 3H_2O + NO + SO_3 + HCl$

10) <u>In diluting an acidic solution for use in the operating theatre, a 6mL solution of 5.0 moles HCl is diluted in 194mL of normal saline. What is its new concentration?</u>

A. 0.6 M

B. 0.15M

C. 0.06M

D. 6.15M

Answers

1) This can be done by eyeballing the point at which the curve goes through its steepest drop. Alternatively, you can mark out at each point along the graph where the aorta sits on the curve, and arteries, and capillaries, etc. Then, measure (using a pen or pencil as a ruler) the distance between each of the answers. The greatest drop occurs between the aorta and the capillaries, so the answer is A.

2) The correct answer is B. This can be calculated as:

A. Length of lever arm is 0.2m (remember that you must correct the units!)

   B. Force applied is 5N

   C. Torque = distance × force

   D. $= 0.2 \times 5 = 1 Nm$ (B)

3) The correct answer is C. This can be worked out as below:

   A. Since the see-saw is balanced, the torque must be equal (otherwise one of the ends would unbalance the other). Thus, since torque on the left (lets call it T_L) must equal torque on the right (lets call it T_R). Since the torques are equal, $T_L = T_R$.

   B. Since torque $= f \times d$, and $T_L = T_R$, then $f_L \times d_L = f_R \times d_R$

   C. This gives you $350 \times 1 = 300 \times d_R$.

   D. From this, $d_R = (350 \times 1)/\, 300 = 350/300 = 1.17m$

4) The correct answer is C. This can be determined by noting that the problem is dilatation of the peripheral arteries and veins, which would most readily be fixed by noradrenaline. Adrenaline is almost the correct answer, but has less effect on the peripheries; plus we are told that the heart is pumping fine, so we do not need any action on the heart (making B incorrect). A and D are incorrect as they have little or negative impact on the peripheral vasculature.

5) The correct answer is D. We worked out above that noradrenaline is the correct drug, so merely use the formula for the noradrenaline dose (0.5–1.5μg/kg/min) for a 75kg male, which is 75 × 0.5 (which gives you the lower range of the dose), and 75 × 1.5 (which gives you the higher range of the dose), and don't forget the units! The answer must contain the units μg/kg/min. A is incorrect as the units are wrong, B is incorrect as this is the dose for dopamine, and C is incorrect as this is the dose for adrenaline. Note how a lot of irrelevant information was given. This is merely to confuse you, as how old he is, his symptoms, his blood pressure and where he works (and so on) are all irrelevant to the question. Ensure you read through quickly (or skip straight to the actual question they are asking), and don't be confused if they give you irrelevant information for a question – as long as you have the information you need to answer, forget about the rest!

6) The correct answer is A. This is a tricky question, as it involves you not only using the given formula, but manipulating it. The answer can be worked out as follows:

A. As the pressures of the two containers are equal, $P_1 = P_2$

B. As $PV = nRT$, then by moving the formula around, $P = (nRT)/V$

C. Since $P_1 = P_2$, then $(n_1R_1T_1)/V_1 = (n_1R_1T_1)/V_1$

D. Working out the P_1 side, $n_1 = 150/(12 + 16 + 16)$, so $n_1 = 3.41$mol (as moles = mass (in grams) divided by molar mass)

E. Substituting in your information for P_1, $P_1 = (3.41 \times 8.314 \times (100 + 273))/5 = (3.41 \times 8.314 \times 373)/5 = 10,575/5 = 2115$ kPa

F. Remember $P_1 = P_2$, so $P_1 = P_2 = 2115 = n_2R_2T_2/V_2$. Substituting in your numbers you have $2115 = (n_2 \times 8.314 \times (273+100))/3$. By moving the formula around, you get $2115 \times 3 = n_2 \times 8.314 \times 373$. This gives you $6345 = 3101 \times n_2$, so $n_2 = 2.046$

G. The formula asked you for the weight of O_2, not the number of moles, so you work this out with $2.046 = \times$ grams of $O_2/32 = 65.4$g

H. As you can see, you must know your chemistry to have any chance at working this out!

7) The answer is D. This is because it *is* possible to make a superimposable mirror image of this molecule. However, it is not possible for the others. Another example of why you need to have a good grasp of chemistry, especially organic chemistry!

8) The correct answer is B. I am afraid the only way you could know this would be to know your organic chemistry very well!

9) The correct answer is C. This is high school chemistry, so would be one of the easier chemistry questions. Equations A, B and D are not balanced, so can be eliminated, while C is.

10) The correct answer is B. This can be calculated as follows:

A. This can be solved simply, by knowing the formula $M_1V_1 = M_2V_2$ (but this requires you to know your chemistry well). Substituting your given values, you get $5 \times 6 = 200 \times Y$ moles, giving you $30 = 200Y$, which gives you 0.15.

B. Therefore, your new concentration is 0.15 moles of HCl

C | Sample Curriculum Vitae

Tom Stewart

Personal Information

Thomas Peter Stewart
123 Border St, Sydney, 2000
0400 000 000
tstewart@zmail.com

Qualifications

Bachelor of Science (Honours 1st Class). Major in Physiology, University of New South Wales, 2007

Certificate IV (Personal Training), 2004

Certificate III (Fitness Instructor), 2004

Higher School Certificate, Karratha High School, New South Wales, 2003

Work History

Orderly, St Elsewhere's Hospital (2008–present)

This entails working closely with patients as part of the healthcare team, including assisting nurses in daily patient care and aiding physiotherapists to increase patient mobility. This role is physically demanding, requires excellent presentation and communication skills, and the ability to work well as part of a team.

Assistant, Elder Consulting (2007–2008)

In assisting with community meetings for a public relations firm, I worked in collaboration with a large team of people from various skill backgrounds, requiring excellent communication and problem solving skills.

Personal Trainer, Tom's Fitness (2004–present)

In 2004 I established a personal training business (ABN 35555555). My goal is to deliver fitness programs that are based on science and enjoyable, to give people the ability to manage their fitness independently.

Awards and Achievements

Summer Research Scholarship (2011), School of Biochemistry, Spurious University

2nd Place – Mid-year Exam (2010), School of Biochemistry, Spurious University

Extra-curricular Activities

Student Mentor – School of Medicine, Sydney (2011)

This involved assisting first year science students with practical and course-related needs as well as social and emotional support, via regular emails and being available if the students wished to get in contact. This required excellent communication and empathy.

Student Liaison and Advocacy, School of Physiology, Spurious University (2007)

This role involved me acting on behalf of the students to voice opinions on course content, teaching methods and assessments. This was a volunteer role, and I was supported both by my fellow students and the academic staff.

Volunteer Work

Volunteer, Sydney Nursing Home (2010)

Every Monday evening and Friday morning I attended the Sydney Nursing Home, spending my time in the Higher Care facilities, assisting with care of patients suffering from dementia. This assisted me in developing skills interacting with and caring for elderly patients, especially patients suffering from degenerative conditions.

Volunteer, Sydney Homeless Shelter (2006–2009)

Every Thursday evening I attended the Sydney Homeless Shelter, and was involved in Youth Outreach and fundraising. This work brought me face to face with those adversely affected by drugs and alcohol, as well as allowed me to develop proactive listening, and practice my communication with difficult subjects.

Referees

Tracey Oakman

Director, Elder Consulting
0405 555 555
toakman@elder.com.au

James Gates

Nurse Unit Manager, St Elsewhere's
Hospital
(02) 7676 7421
james.gates@stelsewheres.com.au

Georgina Thompson

Personal Information

Georgina Thompson
99 Southern Road, Sydney, 2000
0400 050 050
gthompson@hotmail.com

Qualifications

Higher School Certificate, 2011

Chatswood High School, Sydney, New South Wales

ATAR 98.5

Work History

Childcare (2006–current)

This entails being responsible for up to four children between the ages of 2 and 11, up to three times a week. This role involves being high personable, responsible, creative, energetic and organised.

Sales Assistant, Silk, Chatswood (2010–2011)

This role involved customer service duties, including sales ordering stock, opening and closing the boutique, balancing the day's sales and constructively dealing with customer complaints.

Receptionist, St Elsewhere's Clinic (2009–2011)

This involved greeting patients, managing appointments and coordinating visiting doctors. This required being highly organised, well presented, and having effective communication skills in liaising with doctors, other health professionals and patients, and working as part of a team.

Waiter, The Old Hotel, Sydney (2007–2010)

Working at this large establishment involved being responsible for balancing a till, taking food and drink orders as well as managing customer complaints in a professional and constructive manner.

Awards and Achievements

School Captain at Chatswood High School (2011)

Responsible Service of Alcohol Certificate (2010)

The Duke of Edinburgh Bronze, Silver and Gold Awards (2006–2009)

St John's First Aid Certificate (2007)

Surf Life Savings Bronze Medallion (2006)

Extra-curricular Activities

Volunteer, The Retirement Centre, Sydney (2006–2009)

I participated in community service at this hostel twice each week, assisting in conducting co-curricular activities and attending to the residents' needs with compassion and empathy.

Assistant Leader, Kids Outdoor Education Camp Australia (2007–2011)

In this role I acted as an assistant in leading a group of children over a 7-day camp. Working closely with disadvantaged, disabled and troubled children enabled me to develop my active listening skills and practice communicating with various people in challenging situations. As a leader, I was able to develop managerial skills both in interaction with the children, but also with other assisting staff.

Volunteer, Salvation Army Red Shield Appeal (2006)

I provided assistance to the Salvation Army Red Shield Appeal. This involved being highly personable in a one-on-one situation, as well as working effectively in a team environment.

Referees

Keith Shear
Manager
Kids Outdoor Education Camp
Australia
Telephone: (02) 9324 8765
kshear@koeca.com.au

Dr Edward March
Physician
St Elsewhere's Clinic
Telephone: 0450 505 505
edmarch@sec.com.au

D | Interview Questions

Personal Questions

- Why do you want to be a doctor?
- How do you know what it is like to be a doctor?
- What would make you a good doctor?
- What are the downsides to being a doctor? What are the upsides?
- How do you plan to maintain work–life balance?
- What area would you like to get into in medicine?
- What would make you decide to quit medicine?
- If you don't get into medicine what else would you like to do?
- What is something you are proud of achieving?
- What are your strengths?
- What are your weaknesses?
- Who is in your support network? (that is, who do you talk to if you are having problems)
- How do you handle stress?
- Who is your favourite family member and why?
- What role do you play in your group of friends?
- What do you think your mum would say is your best quality?
- What quality is most important in a good doctor – being technically correct, having empathy with your patients, being a good communicator or giving the patient confidence in your judgements? Why?
- What is leadership? Can you give some examples of your leadership experience?
- What makes a good leader?

- What is empathy? Can you give some examples of when your empathy was important?

- What is confidence? Can you give some examples of when you being confident mattered?

- What is teamwork? Can you give some examples of your teamwork?

- What makes a good team member?

- Can you give two examples of problems with team work that you have experienced in the past, and how you resolved these?

- How would you handle a conflict in a team?

- Why is communication important in a team environment?

- What do you know about the university course?

- Why did you apply here rather than one of the other universities?

- How does your philosophy fit with the uni ethos?

- Do you think good health is a strictly biological phenomenon or do you think social factors are a part of good health/well-being? Why do you think this?

- What job do you currently have? Why did you take that job?

- What is the most challenging situation you've been in? How did you deal with this?

- Who is your role model?

- What is a decision you regret making? Why? What would you do differently?

Ethical Questions

- You have a patient with type 2 diabetes who is non-compliant with their treatment regime. What would you say to this patient?

- You have to deliver the news to parents that their baby didn't survive surgery. What would you say?

- A 17-year-old Aboriginal man is admitted to your care in hospital for alcohol poisoning. Who do you think should be involved in his care?

- A Muslim woman is brought into the emergency department where you are the male doctor on duty. You know she is Muslim because she is covered in a black abeya and her face is also covered. She is bleeding profusely.

She is distressed to see that you are the person who is to take care of her and refuses to allow you to touch her. What do you do?

- An elderly man with metastatic bowel cancer comes to you, asking you to prescribe him something that will end his life. What do you say and do?

- What are the major health problems facing Australians? Are these the major health problems facing the Aboriginal community? What are the differences and how do you know this?

- Discuss the pros and cons of abortion.

- What is an ethical situation you may encounter in medicine? How will you deal with it?

- What would you do if a fellow student or doctor appeared depressed or suicidal?

- An 8-year-old Muslim boy has been inadvertently fed a meal of pork while in hospital. The boy is your patient. His father is very angry and upset about this as pork is 'haram' (forbidden). What would you say to him?

- What would you do if you saw a classmate cheat on an exam?

- What are the major ethical issues in medicine today? Choose one of these and tell me why you think this is an important issue for doctors.

- A homeless person has taken to sleeping in the foyer of your building. What do you think about this and what would you do about it?

- Discuss how the government pays for the medical costs of its people.

- What are the major health problems of people who live in rural and remote areas? Do these differ from urban dwellers? If yes, how?

- Do you think people with a mental illness should be treated in psychiatric hospitals, general hospitals, or somewhere else (like at home)? Why?

- Discuss the pros and cons of screening babies for genetic mutations.

- What is the role for preventative medicine?

- At a bus stop, you see a baby in a pram whose mother is smoking a cigarette. What do you do?

- What do you think about the working hours doctors maintain?

- Are there any situations in which children should be taken away from their parents? Is there anything you must consider before doing this?

- You are an intern, and you smell alcohol on the breath of the surgeon heading your team. What do you do?

- How much control should the government have over our health choices?

- You are a GP, and a 15-year-old female patient indicates she is pregnant and wants to have an abortion. What do you do about this request? Her mother calls you to ask about her daughter – what do you tell her?

- You are in a supermarket and you see a young woman with four children who is struggling to manage them. They are behaving badly and in frustration she smacks one of them. What do you do?

- A patient recovering from a heart attack is refusing to have a stent put in one of his coronary arteries, and his wife appeals to you to 'talk some sense into him'. What do you do?

- Why is it important that healthcare professionals are responsible in both their professional and personal lives?

- Should Medicare pay for the care of an obese, alcoholic patient who refuses to quit smoking?

- One of your fellow medical students seems to be struggling with their university work, and seems to be drinking more than usual. What do you do? Is there anyone you would talk to?

- You suspect your neighbour is abusing their child. What do you do?

- What do you think about the amount of medical information available on the internet?

- A patient in a nursing home doesn't want their old prosthetic leg to be replaced with a new one, even though it would be medically best to replace it. The doctor wants to replace it. You are the nurse unit manager – what do you do?

- You are an intern doing some research for your consultant, and he insists you falsify the results. What do you do?

- A businessperson is very stressed at work, and comes to you for sleeping tablets. Do you prescribe the tablets, and what do you say to him/her?

- What are important issues to consider with end of life decisions?

- Discuss the pros and cons of euthanasia.

- Why do many in the community attach a stigma to mental illness?

- Medical school is very competitive, and everyone is extremely bright. How will you feel if you are only an average student?

- Discuss some examples where religion has an impact on medical practice? What do you think of this?

- What are some ways the Australian government could deal with the obesity crisis?

- What are some initiatives to reduce homelessness? What are some of the health problems homeless people suffer?

- Doctors must undergo continuing professional development. What is this? What are the pros and cons of this? Why should doctors do this when most other professions don't?

- A 45-year-old presents unconscious to emergency after a motor vehicle accident, and needs a blood transfusion. A nurse finds a card in their wallet indicating they are a Jehovah's Witness, and wish not to ever have a blood transfusion. What do you do? How would this differ if the patient was 10 years old and his/her parents told you not to transfuse her?

- What are the pros and cons of alternative medicines?

- An 11-year-old female presents to you asking for 'the pill'. What do you do?

- Outline the difference between the public and private healthcare systems.

References

- Australian Indigenous Doctors Association. www.aida.org.au/becoming. aspx

- ANZ Journal of Surgery. *Writing a Curriculum Vitae*. www.anzjsurg.com/ view/0/writingACV.html

- Australian Medical Association. *Becoming a Doctor and Bonded Medical School Places – A Guide for Prospective Medical Students*. http://ama.com.au/ node/4130

- Berndle, A. 2007. *So, You Want to be a Doctor, Eh?* Writing on Stone Press Inc.: Alberta.

- Churchill, J. 2012. 'Internship Uncertainty'. *MJA Insight* 29, 30th July.

- Davenport, C., B. Honigman, J. Druck. 2008. 'The 3-Minute Emergency Medicine Medical Student Presentation: A Variation on a Theme'. *Academic Emergency Medicine* 15: 683–687.

- Dean S., A. Barratt, G. Hendry, P. Lyon. 2003. 'Preparedness for hospital practice amongst graduates of a problem based graduate entry medical program'. *Medical Journal of Australia* 178: 163–167.

- Ellen, S., T. Norman, G. Burrows. 1997. 'Assessment of anxiety and depression in primary care'. *Medical Journal of Australia* 167 (6): 328–333.

- Fritz, D., A. Hu, T. Wilson, H. Ladak, P. Haase, K. Fung. 2011. 'Long-term retention of a 3-dimensional computer model of the larynx'. *Archives of Otolaryngology—Head & Neck Surgery* 137 (6): 598–603.

- Fulde, G. 2012. *Emergency Medicine: The Principles of Practice*, 6th ed. Saunders Australia: Sydney.

- Good Universities Guide. www.gooduniguide.com.au

- Graduate Australian Medical School Admissions Test (GAMSAT) website. www.gamsat-ie.org/gamsat-australia

- Groves, M., J. Gordon, G. Ryan. 2007. 'Entry tests for graduate medical programs: Is it time to rethink?' *Medical Journal of Australia* 186: 120–123.

- Hojat, M., J. Gonnella, S. Mangione, T. Nasca, J. Veloski, J. Erdmann, C. Callahan, M. Magee. 2002. 'Empathy in medical students as related to academic performance, clinical competence and gender'. *Medical Education* 36: 522–527.

- Iyengar, V. 2008. 'Namaste India: Indian women and health'. *O&G Magazine* 10 (2): 16–19.

- Joyce, C., J. Stoelwinder, J. McNeil, L. Piterman. 2003. 'Riding the wave: Current and emerging trends in graduates from Australian university medical schools'. *Medical Journal of Australia* 186 (6): 309–312.

- Koh, G., H. Khoo, M. Wong, D. Koh. 2004. 'The effects of problem-based learning during medical school on physician competency: A systematic review'. *Canadian Medical Association Journal* 178 (1): 34–41.

- Leaders in Indigenous Medical Education. www.limenetwork.net.au

- Mariotti, A. 2009. *Creating Your Teaching Plan: A Guide for Effective Teaching*. AuthorHouse: London.

- Olaitan, A., O. Okunade, J. Corne. 2010. 'How to present clinical cases'. *Student BMJ* 18: c1539.

- ProMed Medical and Dental Student Loans. www.promedfinance.com.au

- Rose, R., B. Schwerdt, M. Jorgensen. 2011. *The Ultimate Resume Guide*. www.seek.com.au/jobs-resources/get-your-dream-job/resume-guide

- Royal Australian College of General Practitioners. www.racgp.org.au

- Royal Australasian College of Physicians. www.racp.edu.au

- Royal Australasian College of Surgeons. www.surgeons.org

- Saltman, D., N. O'Dea, M. Kidd. 2006. 'Conflict management: A primer for doctors in training'. *Graduate Medical Journal* 82 (963): 9–12.

- Sleight, D., B. Mavis. 2009. 'Study Skills and Academic Performance among Second-Year Medical Students in Problem-Based Learning'. *Medical Education Online* 11 (23).

- Smits, P., J. Verbeek, C. de Buisonjé. 2002. 'Problem based learning in continuing medical education: A review of controlled evaluation studies.' *British Medical Journal* 324 (7330): 153–156.

- Sparknotes website. www.sparknotes.com/sparknotes/

- Stewart, M. 1995. 'Effective physician-patient communication and health outcomes: A review'. *Canadian Medical Association Journal* 152 (9): 1423–1433.

- Times Higher Education. *World University Rankings: 2011–12.* www.timeshigherducation.co.uk

- Undergraduate Medicine and Health Sciences Admission Test (UMAT) website. http://umat.acer.edu.au/

- Wilkinson, D., J. Zhang, G. Byrne, H. Luke, I. Ozolins, M. Parker, R. Peterson. 2008. Medical school selection criteria and the prediction of academic performance. *Medical Journal of Australia* 188 (6): 349–354.

Further Reading

Curriculum Vitae Writing and Building, and Interview Skills

- ANZ Journal of Surgery. *Writing a Curriculum Vitae.* www.anzjsurg.com/view/0/writingACV.html

- Duke of Edinburgh's Award website. www.dukeofed.com.au

- Fulde, G. 2012. *Emergency Medicine: The Principles of Practice,* 6th ed. Saunders Australia: Sydney.

- Lloyd, M., R. Bor. 2004. *Communication Skills for Medicine.* Churchill Livingstone: Edinburgh*

- Oliver, V. 2005. *301 Smart Answers to Tough Interview Questions.* Sourcebooks: Naperville, Illinois.

- Rose, R., B. Schwerdt, M. Jorgensen. 2011. *The Ultimate Resume Guide.* www.seek.com.au/jobs-resources/get-your-dream-job/resume-guide

- Seek Volunteer. www.volunteer.com.au

- Toastmasters website. www.toastmasters.org.au

- Youth Volunteering NSW. www.youthvolunteeringnsw.com

Entry to Medical School

- Australian Medical Association. *Becoming a Doctor and Bonded Medical School Places – A Guide for Prospective Medical Students.* http://ama.com.au/node/4130 *

- Australian Medical Students Association. *Premed AMSA. www.amsa.org.au/content/premed-amsa* *

- Berndle, A. 2007. *So, You Want to be a Doctor, Eh?* Writing on Stone Press Inc.: Alberta.*

Medical Ethics

- Breen, K., V. Plueckhahn, S. Cordner. 1997. *Ethics, Law and Medical Practice.* Allen & Unwin: Sydney.*

- Maxwell, B. 2010. *Professional Ethics Education: Studies in Compassionate Empathy.* Springer: North Rhine-Westphalia

- Parker, M., D. Dickenson. 2001. *The Cambridge Medical Ethics Workbook.* Cambridge University Press: Cambridge.*

Medical School Resources

- Davenport, C., B. Honigman, J. Druck. 2008. 'The 3-Minute Emergency Medicine Medical Student Presentation: A Variation on a Theme'. *Academic Emergency Medicine* 15: 683–687.

- Defence Force Scholarships. www.defencejobs.gov.au/education/universitysponsorship/

- John Flynn Placement Program. www.acrrm.org.au/about-john-flynn-placement-program

- McCann, S., E. Wise. 2008. *Anatomy Colouring Book*, 3rd ed. Kaplan Publishing: New York.

- Olaitan, A., O. Okunade, J. Corne. 2010. 'How to present clinical cases'. *Student BMJ* 18: c1539.

- ProMed Medical and Dental Student Loans. www.promedfinance.com.au

- Puggy Hunter Memorial Scholarships. www.rcna.org.au/WCM/RCNA/Scholarships/Government/puggy_hunter/rcna/scholarships/government/puggy_hunter_memorial_scholarship_scheme.aspx

- Royal Australian College of General Practitioners. www.racgp.org.au

- Royal Australasian College of Physicians. www.racp.edu.au

- Royal Australasian College of Surgeons. www.surgeons.org

- Rural Australia Medical Undergraduate Scholarships. http://ramus.ruralhealth.org.au/

- Shem, S. 1980. *The House of God.* Random House; Berkshire.

Medical School Textbooks

- Acland, R. 2003. *Acland's Video Atlas: Set of Six DVDs.* Lippincott Williams & Wilkins: Philadelphia. See also www.aclandanatomy.com

- Boon, N., N. Colledge, B. Walker. 2010. *Davidson's Principles and Practice of Medicine*, 21st ed. Churchill Livingstone: Philadelphia.

- Drake, R. 2009. *Gray's Anatomy for Students*, 2nd ed. Churchill Livingstone: Philadelphia.

- Eizenberg, N., C. Briggs, P. Barker, I. Grkovic. 2012. *Anatomedia*. www.anatomedia.com

- Fauci, A., E. Braunwald, D. Kasper, S. Hauser, D. Longo, J. Jameson, J. Loscalzo. 2011. *Harrison's Principles of Internal Medicine*, 18th ed. McGraw-Hill: New York.

- Fulde, G. 2012. *Emergency Medicine: The Principles of Practice*, 6th ed. Saunders Australia: Sydney.

- Garden, J., A. Bradbury, J. Forsythe, P. Parkes. 2007. *Principles and Practice of Surgery*, 5th ed. Churchill Livingstone: Philadelphia.

- Hall, J. 2011. *Guyton and Hall Textbook of Medical Physiology*, 12th ed. Saunders: Philadelphia.

- Kahn, K. 2008. *Mnemonics and Study Tips for Medical Students*, 2nd ed. Hodder Arnold: London.

- Kumar, P., C. Clark. 2009. *Kumar and Clark's Clinical Medicine*, 7th ed. Saunders: Philadelphia.

- Kumar, V., A. Abbas, N. Fausto. 2009. *Kumar: Robbins and Cotran Pathologic Basis of Disease*, 8th ed. Saunders: Philadelphia.

- Longmore, M., I. Wilkinson, E. Davidson, A. Foulkes, A. Mafi. 2010. *Oxford Handbook of Clinical Medicine*, 8th ed. Oxford University Press: Oxford.

- Marieb, E., K. Hoehn. 2012. *Human Anatomy & Physiology*, 9th ed. Benjamin Cummings: San Francisco.

- Moore, K., A. Dalley, A. Agur. 2009. *Clinically Oriented Anatomy*, 6th ed. Lippincott Williams & Wilkins: Philadelphia.

- Rang, H., M. Dale, J. Ritter, R. Flower. 2011. *Rang and Dale's Pharmacology*, 7th ed. Churchill Livingstone: Philadelphia.

- Sinnatamby, C. 2011. *Last's Anatomy: Regional and Applied*, 12th ed. Churchill Livingstone.

- Smith, S., A. Scarth, M. Sasada. 2011. *Drugs in Anaesthesia and Intensive Care*, 4th ed. Oxford University Press: Oxford.

- Talley, N., S. O'Connor. 2009. *Clinical Examination*, 6th ed. Churchill Livingstone: Sydney.

UMAT, GAMSAT and Study Techniques

- Byron, M. 2008. *The Verbal Reasoning Test Workbook*. Kogan Press; London.

- Chesla, E. 1997. *Reading Skills for College Students*. Prentice Hall; New Jersey.

- Elevate Education. http://au.elevateeducation.com/home

- Graduate Australian Medical School Admissions Test (GAMSAT) website. www.gamsat-ie.org/gamsat-australia.

- Grayling, A. C. 2002. *The Meaning of Things: Applying Philosophy to Life*. Oxford University Press: Oxford.

- Grayling, A. C. 2003. *The Meaning of Things: Living With Philosophy*. Phoenix Paperbacks: Oregon.

- HSC Study website. http://hsc.csu.edu.au/study/

- Kay, P. 1999. *Step by Step Non-verbal Reasoning*. Learning Together; Belfast.

- Langhan, J. 2008. *Improving College Reading Skills*, 5th ed. Townsend Press: New Jersey.

- Maxwell, B. 2010. *Professional Ethics Education: Studies in Compassionate Empathy*. Springer: North Rhine-Westphalia.

- Office of the Qualifications and Examinations Register. http://webarchive.nationalarchives.gov.uk/+/http://www.ofqual.gov.uk/1549.aspx?showEmailForm=true

- Princeton Review. 2011. *Reading and Writing Workout for the SAT*, 2nd ed. Princeton Review: Framingham.

- Sparknotes website. www.sparknotes.com/sparknotes/

- The Official GMAT website. www.mba.com/the-gmat.aspx

- Undergraduate Medicine and Health Sciences Admission Test (UMAT) website. http://umat.acer.edu.au/

Index

Printed in the USA
CPSIA information can be obtained
at www.ICGtesting.com
LVHW041126210924
791747LV00001B/35